Diabetic Neurology

Diabetic Neurology

Douglas W. Zochodne
Department of Clinical Neurosciences
Faculty of Medicine, University of Calgary
Calgary, Alberta, Canada

Gregory Kline
Department of Medicine, Faculty of Medicine
University of Calgary
Calgary, Alberta, Canada

Eric E. Smith
Department of Clinical Neurosciences
Faculty of Medicine, University of Calgary
Calgary, Alberta, Canada

Michael D. Hill
Department of Clinical Neurosciences
Faculty of Medicine, University of Calgary
Calgary, Alberta, Canada

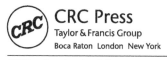

CRC Press
Taylor & Francis Group
Boca Raton London New York

CRC Press is an imprint of the
Taylor & Francis Group, an **informa** business

CRC Press
Taylor & Francis Group
6000 Broken Sound Parkway NW, Suite 300
Boca Raton, FL 33487-2742

First issued in paperback 2017

© 2010 by Taylor & Francis Group, LLC
CRC Press is an imprint of Taylor & Francis Group, an Informa business

No claim to original U.S. Government works

A CIP record for this book is available from the British Library.

Library of Congress Cataloging-in-Publication Data available on application

ISBN-13: 978-1-4200-8553-2 (hbk)
ISBN-13: 978-1-138-11364-0 (pbk)

Typeset by MPS Limited, a Macmillan Company

Visit the Taylor & Francis Web site at
http://www.taylorandfrancis.com

and the CRC Press Web site at
http://www.crcpress.com

This book is dedicated toward our patients with diabetes mellitus in the hope that better care and more effective treatments emerge for them.

Acknowledgment

The authors acknowledge the detailed and timely editorial input by Barbara Zochodne. We also acknowledge the support of the Faculty of Medicine at the University of Calgary and our Departments of Clinical Neurosciences and Medicine. DZ acknowledges the ongoing research support for his work on diabetes that has been provided by the Canadian Institutes of Health Research, the Canadian Diabetes Association, and the Juvenile Diabetes Research Foundation. He is an AHFMR scientist. MH has been funded by the Heart and Stroke Foundation of Alberta/NWT/NU and by Alberta Innovates—Health Solutions. His research has been supported by the CIHR, Heart and Stroke Foundation Alberta/NWT/NU, and the NINDS (NIH). He has received industry support from Hoffmann-La Roche Canada Ltd., Baxter USA, and Merck Canada in the form of drug-in-kind support for clinical trials and salary support for clinical fellows from Bayer Canada.

Dr Smith receives research support from the National Institutes of Neurological Disorders and Stroke, the Canadian Stroke Network, and the Canadian Institutes for Health Research, and salary support from the Canadian Institutes for Health Research.

Contents

Introduction

Diabetologists and neurologists may lead separate but parallel professional lives. Despite some instances of shared clinics and patients, the relationship between these two key subspecialties is rarely appreciated or fully utilized. This is an enormous oversight, particularly in view of the growing global burden of type 2 diabetes mellitus. Consultations involving neurological complications of diabetic patients in the emergency room setting are frequent.

In this book our intent is to bridge the gap between diabetology and neurology with a practitioner-friendly guide for the recognition, investigation, and management of diabetic patients with neurological disease. The goal of our textbook was not to be a comprehensive textual review of diabetic neurological complications, as several excellent examples of these have recently published. We also do not cover detailed pathophysiology or all of the pharmacological considerations in this group of patients. Rather our intent is to provide a comprehensive practical review of the problems encountered at the interface of diabetes and neurology. The point form format facilitates a thorough summary of the diabetological and neurological approach to patients and their related disease states. We address the problems neurologists may encounter in diabetic patients and the important neurological issues to consider in diabetes clinics. The emphasis is on adult patients, and some topics are deliberately covered in more than one section, depending on the context of the discussion.

Section 1 provides overviews of diabetes care directed toward neurologists and of neurological basics directed toward diabetologists. Of interest are abbreviated but comprehensive approaches toward the "full neurological examination," often viewed as a prohibitive and time-consuming process in diabetic clinics. We describe neurological evaluations that can be completed in a timely manner, a cost saving over more expensive forms of testing that may not be necessary. We also show physicians how to expand or tailor their neurological assessments, depending on the patient's history and preliminary findings.

Section 2 provides brief point summaries of a variety of common neurological presentations. We also devote a chapter to "red flags." These are potentially serious issues that both specialties must be cognizant of.

Finally, section 3 highlights specific conditions with significant overlap between diabetes and neurology. Our final chapter presents a grouping of rare conditions, and their neurological and diabetic complications. In particular, this interesting list is expanding with newer associations being recognized yearly.

Diabetic neurology is a growing field in substantial need of increased attention at both the clinical and basic science levels. As one example, the evidence in the literature addressing the efficacy of therapies for stroke and cerebrovascular disease rarely consider diabetic patients as a separate subgroup. The important, direct central nervous system complications of diabetes, including its targeting of white matter, have only been recently recognized. Finally, diabetic neuropathy, more commonly treated in diabetes clinics than neurological clinics, lacks a safe, effective, and inexpensive therapy that arrests or reverses the disorder. Bridging the clinical divide between diabetology and neurology will help.

1

Diabetes basics

In this chapter we outline basic and current information about how diabetes mellitus is diagnosed, evaluated and treated. This information is a starting point for most neurologists who treat diabetic patients.

THE DEFINITION OF DIABETES MELLITUS

KEY POINTS

- Current diagnostic criteria for the definition of diabetes mellitus are endorsed by both the American Diabetes Association (1) and the Canadian Diabetes Association (2).
  - i. Fasting plasma glucose ≥ 7.0 mmol/L (126 mg%) on two occasions OR
  - ii. 75-g oral glucose tolerance test (OGTT) showing a two-hour glucose ≥ 11.1 mmol/L (200 mg%) *or* random plasma glucose ≥ 11.1 mmol/L (200 mg%)
- Recently, the ADA has introduced the concept of HbA1c measurement for diabetes screening; it is possible that this may become the screening test of choice in the near future. A HbA1c > 6.5% (standardized assay reference range 4.3–6.1%) is highly suggestive of a diagnosis of diabetes mellitus.
- The traditional definition of diabetes mellitus was established by epidemiologic studies linking the above criteria with the appearance of diabetic complications.
- Two stages of "prediabetes" are defined as follows:
  - i. Impaired fasting glucose (IFG) [fasting glucose greater than 5.6–6.0 mmol/L but less than 7.0 mmol/L (100–125 mg%)]
  - ii. Impaired glucose tolerance (IGT) [two-hour glucose of 7.8–11.0 mmol/L (140–199 mg%) following 75-g oral glucose load]
  - iii. IFG or IGT may be present separately or together

iv. Both IFG and IGT are associated with a high risk of progression to formal diabetes mellitus

v. Both IFG and IGT are associated with an increased risk of macro-vascular diseases such as ischemic heart disease or stroke

- Diabetes mellitus diagnosed for the first time during pregnancy is termed **gestational diabetes**. Previously undiagnosed type 1 or 2 diabetes may emerge during pregnancy. True gestational diabetes is a separate entity by virtue of the following:

  i. A lack of associated risk for fetal malformations

  ii. The frequent lack of need for pharmacologic/insulin therapy

  iii. Its remission to normal glucose status post partum

  iv. Its prediction of a high future risk for type 2 diabetes

Although frequently recommended in clinical practice guidelines, it is debatable whether the 75-g OGTT is routinely necessary; most diabetics will have an abnormal fasting glucose or HbA1c. Persons with IFG and IGT often fit the clinical picture of "metabolic syndrome" characterized by varying degrees of dyslipidemia, hypertension and obesity. No specific criteria for Metabolic Syndrome are specified here since they vary in the literature. Other than lifestyle measures for diet, exercise and weight loss, there is little outcome-based evidence to support specific long-term pharmacologic glucose-lowering treatments for persons with IFG or IGT. Thus, many experts recommend appropriate treatments for the various components of the Metabolic Syndrome (hypertension, lipids, obesity) along with patient counseling regarding the high future risk of developing frank type 2 diabetes.

ETIOLOGY OF DIABETES MELLITUS

- Diabetes mellitus has traditionally been classified as type 1 or 2 on the basis of age, weight, and presence or absence of ketoacidosis at presentation. However, such factors may have very poor discrimination in both children and adults. A proper diagnosis of diabetes etiology requires long-term follow-up; endocrinology consultation may help to confirm uncertain cases.
- Type 1 diabetes typically refers to insulin deficiency/ketoacidosis prone and may be autoimmune or postpancreatectomy/pancreatitis.
- Type 2 diabetes typically refers to diabetes associated with insulin resistance although insulin deficiency usually develops over time. This is the most common form of diabetes and includes diabetes associated with glucocorticoid use or Cushing's syndrome.
- Rarer forms of secondary diabetes such as hemochromatosis or cystic fibrosis may have features of both types 1 and 2 diabetes.
- Monogenic diabetes—several types of familial diabetes varying from subtle glucose abnormalities to frank insulin requiring diabetes may represent up to 2% to 5% of all diabetics. These individuals may have associated cardiomyopathies, hearing loss, muscle weakness, neonatal

hypoglycemia, renal diseases and other health abnormalities. A family history of autosomal dominant diabetes suggests the diagnosis, prompting genetic testing for confirmation. Also see chapter 17.

SCREENING FOR DIABETES MELLITUS

- Type 2 diabetes may be unrecognized in a significant proportion of the global population. Population screening for diabetes is not discussed here. Individuals presenting with a potential neurologic complication of diabetes should be screened.
- Appropriate screening includes a fasting blood glucose or random blood glucose in the acute care setting.
- The routine use of a two-hour 75-g OGTT is of uncertain value or relevance to patient outcome (3).
- Hemoglobin A1c is not yet recommended for routine screening (see above). In the absence of recent blood loss, it may provide a quantitative estimate of the degree of hyperglycemia in the preceding 120 days. It is an inexpensive and readily available rapid marker for overt diabetes mellitus; false elevations do not occur.
- Specific examples of scenarios recommending diabetes screening in a neurology practice may include
   i. idiopathic sensory polyneuropathy,
   ii. myotonic muscular dystrophy,
   iii. cerebrovascular disease (impact on atherosclerosis risk management),
   iv. mitochondrial disorders (some associated with diabetes; chap. 17),
   v. patients on or about to be treated with glucocorticoids (myasthenia gravis, CIDP, vasculitis, decadron for cerebral edema, others),
   vi. investigation of mononeuropathy/cranial neuropathy, and
   vii. investigation of autonomic dysfunction.

DIABETES FUNCTIONAL REVIEW

- A comprehensive diabetes assessment may be time consuming if all pertinent questions and examinations are completed. A general mnemonic (DCCT, in honor of the landmark trial (4)) is proposed to assist with an organized assessment.
   i. Diagnosis
      i. How diagnosed? When?
      ii. Familial component?
      iii. Does the story fit a classic type 1 or 2 pattern?
   ii. Control
      i. Is glucose monitoring being done?
         a. Does patient self-interpret results or self-adjust medications?
         b. Are hemoglobin A1c measures being done? What is the long-term trend in HbA1c results?

    ii. What drug therapy is employed?
      a. Insulin—types, frequency, sites
      b. Oral agents—adherence, side effects, costs
   iii. How frequently does hypoglycemia occur?
      a. Does the patient know what precipitates hypoglycemia?
      b. Is a "medic alert" bracelet being used?
      c. Has hypoglycemia unawareness developed?
      d. How is motor vehicle operation or occupation been impacted?
iii. Complications
   i. Macrovascular
      a. Signs/symptoms of TIA/stroke
      b. Signs/symptoms of angina/heart failure
      c. Resistant hypertension (renovascular)
      d. Peripheral claudication?
   ii. Microvascular
      a. Ophthalmology examinations? Retinopathy?
      b. Renal disease/screening for albuminuria
      c. Neurologic symptoms (*Although many diabetic complications have traditionally been labeled "microvascular," recent work on pathogenesis, especially of neuropathy, argues against microvascular disease as the primary trigger.*)
         i. Sensory loss
        ii. Muscle wasting
       iii. Foot infections/ulceration
       iv. Chronic pain
        v. Excessive sweating
       vi. Postural hypotension
      vii. Erectile dysfunction
     viii. Infertility (retrograde ejaculation)
       ix. Gastroparesis/satiety
        x. Diarrhea, especially nocturnal
   iii. Associations
      a. Dyslipidemia screening/treatment
      b. Hypertension screening/treatment
      c. Sleep apnea screening
      d. Autoimmune thyroid disease/celiac/adrenal
iv. *Te*achable issues
   i. Lifestyle
      a. Smoking cessation
      b. Weight management
      c. Ethanol use
      d. Social/financial stressors
      e. Psychiatric comorbidities
   ii. Self-understanding of
      a. metabolic targets
      b. medication effects
      c. hypoglycemia/hyperglycemia prevention

iii. Fertility
    a. Glycemic control before pregnancy
    b. Risks in other diabetic family members

DIABETIC PHYSICAL EXAMINATION

- Diabetes mellitus or its complications may involve all parts of the body. A complete physical examination is required, with special attention to the following, again using the "DCCT" mnemonic:
  - i. *D*iagnosis
    - i. Cushingoid features (moon facies, plethora, skin thinning, bruising, striae, proximal muscle weakness)?
    - ii. Hemochromatosis (bronze skin colouration)?
    - iii. Body habitus: BMI/waist circumference
    - iv. Presence of signs of insulin resistance (skin tags, acanthosis nigricans)
  - ii. *C*ontrol
    - i. Insulin administration sites—lipohypertrophy/lipoatrophy
  - iii. *C*omplications
    - i. Vital signs, presence of postural hypotension, lack of postural increase in heart rate
    - ii. Direct funduscopy—retinopathy/hemorrhage/neovascularization
    - iii. Cranial nerve examination (see chap. 2)
    - iv. Mouth—dental caries/gingivitis
    - v. Thyroid (goitre?)
    - vi. Carotid, renal, femoral bruits
    - vii. Peripheral sensory examination (may include monofilament; see chap. 2)
    - viii. Peripheral motor examination (see chap. 2)
    - ix. Inspection of feet (deformity, ulcer, infection, skin breakdown, pulses)
  - iv. "*T*ricky" tests
    - i. Gastric succession splash (delayed gastric emptying)
    - ii. Valsalva maneuvre (loss of postrelaxation bradycardia in cardiac autonomic neuropathy)
    - iii. Testicular examination (diabetes-associated hypogonadism)

A PRIMER ON ANTIDIABETIC MEDICATIONS

- Many pharmacologic options are available for lowering blood glucose and new approaches are in development. The choice of agent may be complex. Considerations include drug efficacy, effect on long-term clinical outcomes, safety, cost, side effect profile, frequency of dosing, and interaction with other agents in use. There are few adequately powered long-term outcome studies with single agents or comparisons of pharmaceutical options beyond one to two years. Global clinical practice guidelines (5,6) frequently focus on traditional therapies such as metformin, sulfonylureas and insulin as first line while other agents are classified as optional second line agents, pending more long-term data and cost considerations.

- Metformin (maximum dose 2500 mg, usually divided b.i.d.).
  i. Mechanism of action uncertain; decreases hepatic gluconeogenesis
  ii. Inexpensive, b.i.d. dosing [more expensive long-acting once-daily (o.d.) dosing available]
  iii. Generally lowers HbA1c by around 1% (much greater effect if used for initial monotherapy)
  iv. Not associated with weight gain or hypoglycemia
  v. May be associated with nausea, GI upset
  vi. Possibly implicated (controversial) in the very rare appearance of type B lactic acidosis—not used in renal insufficiency
  vii. UKPDS study suggested a beneficial decrease in cardiac events with metformin in an obese subgroup (7)
- Sufonylureas (Glyburide, Gliclazide, Glimepiride, Glibenclamide).
  i. Action is to increase pancreatic insulin secretion
  ii. Inexpensive, usually o.d. or b.i.d. dosing
  iii. Generally lowers HbA1c by around 1% but may lose efficacy with progressive islet cell failure in type 2 diabetes
  iv. Possible hypoglycemia risk
  v. Modest weight gain with long-term use is common
- Meglitinides (Repaglinide, Nateglinide).
  i. Insulin secretagogue acting through a different receptor than sulfonylureas
  ii. Shorter half-life, usually requires t.i.d.-meal dosing
  iii. Possibly less effective than sulfonylureas at lowering HbA1c despite better control of postprandial glucose; not for use in combination with sulfonylureas (not additive)
  iv. More expensive than sulfonylureas
  v. Can cause hypoglycemia, may be associated with some weight gain with longer term use
  vi. Hepatic metabolism, theoretically safer than sulfonylureas in advanced renal insufficiency
  vii. No long-term outcome studies
- α-Glucosidase inhibitors (Acarbose).
  i. Inhibits/delays postmeal glucose absorption in small bowel, decreases postprandial glucose peak
  ii. Modest cost, usually used t.i.d. with meals
  iii. Small effect upon lowering HbA1c, usually <0.5% change
  iv. Not associated with hypoglycemia or weight gain
  v. Use is usually very limited by severe flatulence, diarrhea, GI upset
  vi. Possible reduction in "conversion" to type 2 diabetes among users with IFG/IGT but no long-term clinical outcome studies (8)

- Thiazolidenediones (TZD; Rosiglitazone, Pioglitazone).
  i. PPAR-γ agonists—multiple mechanisms of action including increased differentiation of adipocytes, up-regulation of factors important for insulin signal transduction—thus traditionally called "insulin sensitizers"
  ii. Brand name versions are expensive relative to other diabetes options
  iii. o.d. dosing but full effect may take up to three months
  iv. Modest effect on HbA1c around 0.5% to 1.0%
  v. Additive effect to other hypoglycemia medications
  vi. Commonly associated with weight gain, edema
  vii. Less frequent associations with congestive heart failure, macular edema, osteoporosis, fractures
  viii. While controversial, a possible increase in cardiac disease/heart failure and deaths with rosiglitazone has been described (9,10)
  ix. No evidence of significant long-term clinical benefits on outcomes despite promising changes in surrogate markers (HbA1c, microalbuminuria)
- Incretin therapies.
  i. Glucagon-like peptide (GLP)-1 agonists (Amylin)
    i. Meal-stimulated increase in insulin secretion; delayed gastric emptying/glucose absorption
    ii. Short-acting agent, requires subcutaneous (SC) injection prior to meals although longer-acting forms in development
    iii. May potentiate hypoglycemia with sulfonylurea or insulin use
    iv. Modest reductions in HbA1c usually <1%
    v. Not associated with weight gain but may cause significant nausea
    vi. No long-term outcome studies
    vii. Currently not widely available
  ii. Dipeptidyl peptidase (DPP)-4 inhibitors (Sitagliptin, Vildagliptin)
    i. Inhibits enzyme that catabolizes GLP-1
    ii. Oral agent, usually o.d. dosing
    iii. More expensive than many other oral agents
    iv. Side effects/efficacy are similar to GLP-1 agonists; may also have immunsuppressive actions predisposing patients to upper respiratory tract infections
    v. No long-term outcome studies

A PRIMER ON INSULIN PRODUCTS

- A detailed review of insulin use is beyond the scope of this primer; brief guidelines are described here.
- Virtually all insulin products used in North America today are human insulins or modified insulin analogues given subcutaneously. Animal insulins are no longer used. Insulin use differs from other forms of pharmacotherapy. Insulin requires individualized, regular assessment and adjustment

to dosing regimens. It is required for all type 1 diabetic persons. The majority of persons with type 2 diabetes will eventually require insulin if they are to achieve some degree of near-normal glycemic control. When insulin therapy requires more than two injections per day, consultation with a general internist/endocrinologist or diabetes nurse educator is recommended.

- Human long-acting insulins (Humulin N or Novolin NPH).
    i. Usually given at bedtime, sometimes in a.m. as well.
    ii. Sometimes an unpredicatable action—onset of hypoglycemic effect at 3 to 5 hours post injection, peak effect at 6 to 10 hours post injection and waning of effect at 12 to 18 hours post injection.
    iii. Most common "first step" in insulin initiation in type 2 diabetes—8 to 10 units at bedtime to control fasting blood glucose.
    iv. All insulins may be associated with hypoglycemia, weight gain, and, rarely, fluid retention/edema/pulmonary edema. True insulin allergy is extremely rare with human insulins.
- Human short-acting insulins [Humulin Regular (Humulin R) or Novolin Toronto].
    i. Usually administered with or prior to a meal.
    ii. Variable clinical effect—onset of effect at one hour post injection, peak effect around two to four hours post injection and waning of effect at four to six hours post injection.
    iii. Usually taken from once to three times per day as required to control daytime glycemia.
- Long-acting insulin analogues (insulin glargine, insulin detemir).
    i. Slight structure change in insulin molecule allows slow dissociation from injection depot at relatively constant rate.
    ii. Similar in unit for unit potency to human long-acting insulins.
    iii. More expensive than human insulin.
    iv. Some patients may experience 24 hours duration of effect but b.i.d. dosing still commonly required.
    v. Slightly fewer nocturnal hypoglycemic episodes compared with long-acting human insulins in type 1 diabetes.
    vi. Consistent dose by dose effect may allow more aggressive dose titration but there is very little data to prove superiority to human long-acting insulins in glycemic control.
- Short-acting insulin analogues (insulin lispro, aspart, glulisine).
    i. Slight modification to insulin structure permits more rapid absorption from SC depot.
    ii. Similar in overall potency to short-acting human insulins, slightly more expensive.
    iii. Onset of action usually 10 to 15 minutes, peak at 30 to 60 minutes, and waning of effect from 1.5 to 4 hours.
    iv. May provide better control of postprandial glucose than human short-acting insulin.

    v. Typically used in the multiple daily injection (MDI) therapy and insulin pumps in combination with dose formulas for carbohydrate intake and "corrections."
- Insulin pumps.
  - i. 24-hour continuous subcutaneous insulin infusion (CSII) using exclusively short-acting insulin analogues.
  - ii. Highly individualizable, programmable insulin delivery rates.
  - iii. Intensive insulin micromanagement may be the best option for very tight glycemic control. Success in glycemic control very user-dependent, not necessarily better than standard MDI therapy.
  - iv. Labor intensive for user, requires six to eight or more glucose tests per day.
  - v. Costly, currently around C$6000 to purchase the insulin pump not including costs of C$300/mo in pump supplies.
  - vi. Risk of diabetic decompensation from unrecognized pump failure.
- Premixed insulin therapies (30/70, 50/50, Mix 25, etc.).
  - i. Convenient means of combining short and long-acting insulin therapies without multiple injections.
  - ii. May improve glycemic control when MDI therapy is not accepted or feasible.
  - iii. Very limited ability to adjust dose since two types of insulin present.
  - iv. Lack of day-to-day adjustability limits its usefulness compared with MDI.

CONTROL OF HYPERGLYCEMIA

Glycemic Control of Outpatients

- Glucose control on a day-to-day basis is a dynamic effort that must take into account meal timing, size and carbohydrate content, both planned and unplanned exercise, sleep/wake cycle, occupation, hypoglycemia prevention, patient understanding and finally motivation and regular self-assessment of the results being achieved. This process is complex, especially in the setting of other medical illness or competing social stressors/demands. Where possible, diabetes management should be conducted through a multidisciplinary clinic where regular follow-up can be achieved and education given.
- Clinical Practice Guidelines suggest a target HbA1c of <7.0% based on the DCCT and UKPDS trials. In type 1 diabetes, better control is linked to fewer diabetic complications throughout life. However, tight glycemic control in type 2 diabetes is more controversial following the publications of ADVANCE (11), VADT (12), and ACCORD (13), all major trials where tight glycemic control (compared with good, but less tight control) failed to alter disease progression/event rates in type 2 diabetes. Therefore, it is difficult at this time to choose a single glycemic target on the basis of

current evidence. Expert endocrinologist opinion advises a philosophy of targeting the best glycemic control that is reasonably attainable, without neglecting the equal importance of issues such as hypoglycemia, hypertension, dyslipidemia, cost management and avoidance of polypharmacy.

Glycemic Control of Inpatients

- There is a high prevalence of diabetes mellitus among hospitalized patients. Inpatient diabetes control is complicated by different meal content and schedules, lack of activity/immobilization, acute stress and illness, medications, infections and other factors. There is limited data proving that tight glycemic control outside of the ICU or CCU makes a significant difference to survival but it may have a role in acute vascular events, ability to heal infections and duration of hospital stay. Medical or Endocrinology consultation may be helpful for such management. Two basic principles are as follows:
    i. Frequent (usually QID) monitoring of capillary blood glucose. It is essential to have adequate and clear glycemic data to evaluate and care for the sick or unstable diabetic patient.
    ii. Emphasis on short-acting insulin use. Oral agents are generally of limited value in a sick or unstable diabetic person. Frequent short-acting insulin use is valuable when potentially rapid changes in medical status or glucose control are occurring.
    iii. Avoidance of the "insulin sliding scale" in most patients. Although convenient and widely used, the sliding scale is associated with poorer diabetes control and longer hospital stays than insulin which is ordered and adjusted daily proactively (14). If the sliding scale is used, it should be limited in scope so that poor control can be recognized.

Glycemic Control in the Unstable Neurology Patient

- From a diabetes management standpoint, instability is defined as hemodynamic compromise, an unresponsive or fluctuating level of consciousness (LOC), rapid (or potential for rapid) change in medical condition, and prolonged NPO status.
- For unstable patients, especially ketosis-prone (type 1) diabetes, the use of intravenous (IV) insulin infusions is recommended if it can be administered in a highly monitored setting. There is debate in the literature regarding the need to achieve "normoglycemia" with IV insulin but IV insulin is the easiest way to achieve and maintain some degree of glycemic control in the unstable diabetic patient for whom the risk of decompensation is great (15).
- IV insulin is typically ordered as 50 units of Regular/Toronto in 500 cc of D5W (= 1 unit/10 cc). The IV tubing should be flushed with 50 cc of this

solution to saturate any insulin binding to the tubing surface. The infusion can then be started at one to two units/hr and increased or decreased in increments of one to two units/hr on the basis of hourly capillary glucose monitoring. The half-life of IV insulin is approximately four to five minutes, which allows for rapid titration guided by meticulous hourly glucose monitoring for safety. With this approach, it is possible to safely maintain glucose levels below 10 mmol/L.

Glycemic Control in Special Neurology Ward Situations

- Continuous tube feeding or parenteral nutrition (i.e., poststroke, motor neuron disease, etc.). These patients pose a challenge for glycemic control by requiring nutrition administration at schedules other than three times daily.
  i. If feeds are intermittent (i.e., q6 hourly over 24 hours) or continuous (hourly), a typical starting order would be Regular insulin sc q6h with feeds. Since the duration of action of regular insulin is about six hours, it is not usually necessary to add a long-acting insulin. In the severely insulin resistant/obese patient, the addition of b.i.d. NPH may be particularly useful with continuous hourly feeds.
  ii. Special care is essential in this setting as feeding amounts and durations/frequencies are often altered by the clinical nutrition teams. If the insulin is not concomitantly adjusted, severe hypo or hyperglycemia may result.
  iii. In particularly difficult cases, it may be useful to provide an IV insulin drip, adjusted to hourly capillary glucose measurements over 24 hours to establish total 24-hour insulin requirements. This total amount may then be given in q6 hourly divided doses and then further titrated to effect.
- Glucocorticoid-induced diabetes (also see chap. 2).
  iv. Supraphysiologic glucocorticoids (more than 7.5 mg/day prednisone or its equivalent) increase overall insulin resistance and increase lipolysis which acts as substrate for gluconeogenesis. This may cause a generalized increase in glycemia although the "classic" response is a progressive rise in glucose levels throughout the day, especially following meals.
  v. Ensure glucose is checked regularly before meals to assess hyperglycemia; most patients will require daily insulin adjustment until stable.
  vi. α-Glucosidase inhibitors, such as TZD, are not helpful agents for steroid induced diabetes because of their very modest glucose-lowering actions and slow onset (with TZD)
  vii. Short-acting insulin with meals is typically required and is the easiest to adjust as necessary. Agents like metformin and sulfonylureas may be useful in relative mild hyperglycemia but are more difficult to adjust on a daily basis.

viii. Careful attention to insulin doses is necessary during glucocorticoid down-titration or cessation to avoid hypoglycemia.

Insulin Dosing in the Insulin-Naïve Patient

- There is no single correct dose or regimen of insulin for individuals with diabetes. Textbook formulae for 24-hour insulin regimens are rarely accurate, and do not apply to treatment of type 2 diabetes.
- For the insulin requiring patient, insulin serves two purposes.
  i. To stop/prevent lipolysis leading to ketoacidosis in a type 1, ketosis-prone diabetic patient. This is of immediate medical importance but *does not always require that hyperglycemia be immediately and fully corrected and prevented.* Except in severe decompensation, it requires less insulin to stop lipolysis than it does to lower blood glucose. Since euglycemia is not required to prevent or arrest ketoacidosis, when starting insulin in the *stable*, insulin-*naïve* patient, even if ketosis prone, it is acceptable to begin with a "safe" lower dose. At the outset the insulin dose required for rapid euglycemia may be impossible to predict. Doses of NPH 6 to 10 units b.i.d. or R insulin 4 to 6 units t.i.d. meals are appropriate initial doses—further dose escalation can quickly be made in response to glucose testing results.
  ii. Control carbohydrate associated hyperglycemia: Depending on the amount of carbohydrate intake, its rate of absorption and insulin resistance, a larger dose of insulin than normally required to prevent lipolysis/acidosis is needed. Acute (often postprandial) hyperglycemia without lipolysis or ketosis is rarely an urgent problem unless it is a recurrent feature of very poor chronic control. Identification of acute ketoacidosis is important during acute hyperglycemia: Confirm with a urine dip for ketones or a measurement of plasma anion gap. If either urine ketones or anion gap exists with hyperglycemia, more aggressive insulin therapy is required immediately.
- For the patient who is *chronically* using insulin and requires hospitalization, a drastic reduction of insulin dose should be avoided despite reduced intake. Small reductions of insulin doses, especially ultra-short-acting meal doses, can be considered although the acute stress of illness, immobilization and infection all increase insulin resistance and gluconeogenesis, often off-setting the lack of oral glucose intake. Large reductions in insulin doses are usually met with marked hyperglycemia. Frequent capillary glucose monitoring and insulin dose readjustment will allow appropriate titration and prevent miscalculation.

2

Neurological basics

This chapter reviews essential features of the neurological evaluation and neurological tests likely to be useful in diabetic patients. Several forms of "screening" evaluation are presented. The information is directed particularly toward diabetologists and diabetologists in training and is a useful refresher for neurologists.

KEY POINTS

- An appropriate and tailored neurological examination is appropriate for busy diabetes clinics and can be carried out rapidly.
- It is cost-effective to perform a clinical neurological examination before ordering specific neurological investigations; investigations not well chosen may delay the diagnosis.
- A systematic approach involving mental status, speech, cranial nerves, motor function, reflexes, sensory examination, and gait is preferred.
- Several screening neurological examinations are available for specific problems or symptoms: for polyneuropathy, autonomic screening, focal neuropathies, hemiparesis, dementia.
- Neurological investigations should be tailored toward the working diagnosis and clinical evaluation.
- Routine use of imaging studies for all neurological problems in diabetic patients may not be sensitive or cost-effective.

REVIEW OF THE NEUROLOGICAL HISTORY (NEUROLOGICAL FUNCTIONAL INQUIRY)

Ask About the Following Problems

- Head, neck, back, or limb trauma; neurosurgical procedures
- Headaches (quality, onset, severity, frequency, location, timing, impact of treatment)

- History of a previous neurological infection (e.g., meningitis, poliomyelitis, encephalitis)
- Visual loss, diplopia, drooping eyelids, childhood squint, positive visual symptoms (flashing lights, lightning bolts, sparkles), light intolerance, transient loss of vision
- Difficulties with hearing, tasting, smelling, chewing, swallowing (choking on solids or liquids); tinnitus; abnormal tastes or smells
- Dizziness, vertigo (a true sensation of self or environment spinning)
- Numbness (loss of sensation), tingling, prickling, "pins and needles," tightness, shooting electrical sensations or burning pain, other types of pain
- Loss of muscle, cramping or twitching muscles (including fasciculations—irregular contractions of parts of muscles), other abnormal movements (e.g., tremor), muscle weakness, incoordination, clumsiness, dragging of leg or foot
- Bowel and bladder—sensation to fullness, ability to empty, incontinence
- Gait—unsteady, falling, dragging limb, difficulty going up or downstairs

NEUROLOGICAL EXAMINATION

When to Do a Full Neurological Examination or Simpler, Abbreviated Version

- A full examination is indicated for new neurological problems, when neurological referral is anticipated and prior to neurological investigations such as nerve conduction or imaging.
- An abbreviated neurological examination can be done for screening to decide if there is a neurological problem or to follow up on a neurological problem.
- An abbreviated neurological examination needs only 5 to 10 minutes. Table 2.1 lists a summary of the key parts of an abbreviated examination and suggestions on how it can be expanded as necessary.

How to Do an Abbreviated but Comprehensive Neurological Examination (5–10 minutes)

- A systematic approach is recommended: top to bottom mental status, cranial nerves, motor examination (including coordination), deep tendon reflexes, sensation, gait, and stance.
- The patient must be dressed in an examining gown or equivalent to do a proper neurological examination.

Mental Status

A normal mental status can be largely identified during the patient interview. Formal testing is required if the patient or witness is specifically complaining

Table 2.1 Summary of the Neurological Examination

What part?	How to do it?	What is normal?
Mental status	Talk with the patient (add formal tests: orientation, calculation, spell WORLD backward, interpret proverbs, MoCA)	Normal insight, memory, ability to describe
Speech	Repeat, enunciate (add reading, writing, naming, pahpahpahtahtahtahkahkahkah)	Repeats normally, no slurring of speech (dysarthria)
Cranial nerves	II–XII: visual fields, pupils, examination of the fundi, extraocular movements, facial movement and sensation, palate and tongue movement, shoulder abduction (add visual acuity, olfaction (I), taste, tongue power, gag reflex, jaw jerk)	No loss of vision or field deficit; normal pupillary reaction; no retinopathy; symmetric facial, palate, and tongue movement Normal sensation in all three divisions of fifth nerve
Motor	Bulk, power (choose a distal and a proximal muscle in each limb), tone, coordination (FNF test, HS test), check for drift of outstretched hands, abnormal movement (add additional muscles in the limb where the problem is and compare with contralateral, other tests of coordination)	No wasting, weakness, rigidity, spasticity, tremor, other abnormal movements, incoordination; no pronator drift of the outstretched hands
Reflexes	Biceps, triceps, brachioradialis, quadriceps (knee), gastrocnemius (ankle), plantar responses	Symmetrical, elicited without reinforcement; plantars are downgoing
Sensation	Light touch, pinprick, cold, vibration, toe position (add 2-point discrimination, warm sensation, direction of movement on the skin)	No change distal (fingers, toes) to proximal; right to left are comparable; vibration present in the toes
Gait and stance	Normal walking, tandem walking (heel to toe), standing on toes, heels; check for a Romberg sign (add a "sharpened" Romberg, arising from a squat)	No evidence of hemiparesis, steppage gait, spasticity, other abnormalities

Additional tests as needed.

Abbreviations: MoCA, Montreal Cognitive Assessment; FNF, finger-nose-finger; HS, heel-shin.

about a change in behavior or memory. The preferred assessment is the MoCA (Montreal Cognitive Assessment) provided in Table 2.2.

Speech

Normal speech may also be identified during the interview. There are two considerations when examining speech. Both can be checked rapidly as follows:

- *Speech articulation*: Abnormalities of articulation are called dysarthria (slurring of speech). Dysarthria can usually be identified during the history by simply listening to the patient speak. More specifically, ask the patient to say pahpahpahpah (lips), tahtahtahtah (tongue), kahkahkahkah (palate) or "Royal Irish Constabulary."
- *Language function*: There are six basic aspects to testing language: (*i*) naming, (*ii*) repetition, (*iii*) fluency, (*iv*) comprehension, (*v*) reading, and (*vi*) writing. Many are tested informally during history taking. Ask the patient to repeat a sentence (e.g., "No ifs, ands, or buts"). This tests comprehension (receptive speech area, temporal lobe), speech motor output (expressive speech area, frontal lobe), and the cortical connections between these parts of the brain [superior longitudinal fasciculus (also known as arcuate fasciculus)]. The patient can also be asked to name or identify objects and read and write a sentence.

Cranial Nerves

These are important to examine systematically from I to XII. In practice olfaction, mediated by the first cranial nerve (I), is not commonly tested (systematic testing of olfaction, however, may be useful in the early prediction of some neurodegenerative disorders).

- For *II*, there are four basic components: (*i*) visual acuity, (*ii*) visual fields, (*iii*) pupillary reflexes, and (*iv*) direct funduscopy. Check the visual fields by confrontation (counting fingers in each quadrant close to the center of the field, but not out in the peripheral vision; wiggling fingers is less sensitive than simply asking the patient to count fingers). Next have the patient cover each eye in turn and look at the examiner's face (ask, "Can you see all of my face?"). A scotoma is an area of missing vision or visual loss. Examine for pupil reactivity to light (done in a darkened room) and to accommodation (watch the pupils as your finger moves from the distance to just in front of the nose). Check for overall pupil size and symmetry. Look for ptosis (drooping of upper lid). Funduscopic examination is a mandatory part of the neurological examination. Color vision, image distortion, and depth perception are special types of visual assessment and may be considered under special circumstances.

(*Text continued on page 22*)

Table 2.2 Montreal Cognitive Assessment Tool

MONTREAL COGNITIVE ASSESSMENT (MOCA)

NAME :
Education :   Date of birth :
Sex :   DATE :

VISUOSPATIAL / EXECUTIVE

Copy cube

Draw CLOCK (Ten past eleven)
(3 points)

POINTS

(E) End   (A)
(5)
(1) Begin   (B)   (2)
(D)   (4)
(3)
(C)

[ ]

[ ]

[ ] Contour   [ ] Numbers   [ ] Hands

__/5

NAMING

[ ]   [ ]   [ ]   __/3

MEMORY Read list of words, subject must repeat them. Do 2 trials, even if 1st trial is successful. Do a recall after 5 minutes.

		FACE	VELVET	CHURCH	DAISY	RED	
	1st trial						No points
	2nd trial						

ATTENTION Read list of digits (1 digit/ sec.).

Subject has to repeat them in the forward order   [ ] 2 1 8 5 4
Subject has to repeat them in the backward order   [ ] 7 4 2   __/2

Read list of letters. The subject must tap with his hand at each letter A. No points if ≥ 2 errors

[ ] F B A C M N A A J K L B A F A K D E A A A J A M O F A A B   __/1

Serial 7 subtraction starting at 100   [ ] 93   [ ] 86   [ ] 79   [ ] 72   [ ] 65   __/3

4 or 5 correct subtractions: **3 pts**, 2 or 3 correct: **2 pts**, 1 correct: **1 pt**, 0 correct: **0 pt**

LANGUAGE Repeat : I only know that John is the one to help today. [ ]
The cat always hid under the couch when dogs were in the room. [ ]   __/2

Fluency / Name maximum number of words in one minute that begin with the letter F   [ ] _____ (N ≥ 11 words)   __/1

ABSTRACTION Similarity between e.g. banana - orange = fruit   [ ] train – bicycle   [ ] watch - ruler   __/2

DELAYED RECALL

Has to recall words WITH NO CUE	FACE [ ]	VELVET [ ]	CHURCH [ ]	DAISY [ ]	RED [ ]	Points for UNCUED recall only	__/5
Optional Category cue							
Multiple choice cue							

ORIENTATION [ ] Date   [ ] Month   [ ] Year   [ ] Day   [ ] Place   [ ] City   __/6

© Z.Nasreddine MD   Version 7.1   **www.mocatest.org**   Normal ≥ 26 / 30   TOTAL   __/30

Administered by: _____   Add 1 point if ≤ 12 yr edu

(continued)

Table 2.2   Montreal Cognitive Assessment Tool (*Continued*)

Montreal Cognitive Assessment
(MoCA)

Administration and Scoring Instructions

The Montreal Cognitive Assessment (MoCA) was designed as a rapid screening instrument for mild cognitive dysfunction. It assesses different cognitive domains: attention and concentration, executive functions, memory, language, visuoconstructional skills, conceptual thinking, calculations, and orientation. Time to administer the MoCA is approximately 10 minutes. The total possible score is 30 points; a score of 26 or above is considered normal.

1.   **Alternating Trail Making:**
          Administration: The examiner instructs the subject: *"Please draw a line, going from a number to a letter in ascending order. Begin here* [point to (1)] *and draw a line from 1 then to A then to 2 and so on. End here* [point to (E)]."

          Scoring: Allocate one point if the subject successfully draws the following pattern:
1 –A- 2- B- 3- C- 4- D- 5- E, without drawing any lines that cross. Any error that is not immediately self-corrected earns a score of 0.

2.   **Visuoconstructional Skills (Cube):**
          Administration: The examiner gives the following instructions, pointing to the **cube**:   *"Copy this drawing as accurately as you can, in the space below".*

          Scoring: One point is allocated for a correctly executed drawing.
          • Drawing must be three-dimensional
          • All lines are drawn
          • No line is added
          • Lines are relatively parallel and their length is similar (rectangular prisms are accepted)
          A point is not assigned if any of the above-criteria are not met.

3.   **Visuoconstructional Skills (Clock):**
          Administration: Indicate the right third of the space and give the following instructions: *"Draw a* **clock***. Put in all the numbers and set the time to 10 after 11".*

          Scoring: One point is allocated for each of the following three criteria:
          ▪ Contour (1 pt.):   the clock face must be a circle with only minor distortion acceptable (e.g., slight imperfection on closing the circle);
          ▪ Numbers (1 pt.): all clock numbers must be present with no additional numbers; numbers must be in the correct order and placed in the approximate quadrants on the clock face; Roman numerals are acceptable; numbers can be placed outside the circle contour;
          ▪ Hands (1 pt.): there must be two hands jointly indicating the correct time; the hour hand must be clearly shorter than the minute hand; hands must be centred within the clock face with their junction close to the clock centre.
          A point is not assigned for a given element if any of the above-criteria are not met.

MoCA Version November 12, 2004
© *Z. Nasreddine MD*

Table 2.2 (*Continued*)

4.   <u>**Naming:**</u>

<u>Administration</u>: Beginning on the left, point to each figure and say: *"Tell me the name of this animal"*.

<u>Scoring</u>: One point each is given for the following responses: (1) camel or dromedary, (2) lion, (3) rhinoceros or rhino.

5.   <u>**Memory:**</u>

<u>Administration</u>: The examiner reads a list of 5 words at a rate of one per second, giving the following instructions: *"This is a memory test. I am going to read a list of words that you will have to remember now and later on. Listen carefully. When I am through, tell me as many words as you can remember. It doesn't matter in what order you say them"*. Mark a check in the allocated space for each word the subject produces on this first trial. When the subject indicates that (s)he has finished (has recalled all words), or can recall no more words, read the list a second time with the following instructions: *"I am going to read the same list for a second time. Try to remember and tell me as many words as you can, including words you said the first time."* Put a check in the allocated space for each word the subject recalls after the second trial.

At the end of the second trial, inform the subject that (s)he will be asked to recall these words again by saying, *"I will ask you to recall those words again at the end of the test."*

<u>Scoring</u>: No points are given for Trials One and Two.

6.   <u>**Attention:**</u>

<u>Forward Digit Span: Administration</u>: Give the following instruction: *"I am going to say some numbers and when I am through, repeat them to me exactly as I said them"*. Read the five number sequence at a rate of one digit per second.

<u>Backward Digit Span: Administration</u>: Give the following instruction: *"Now I am going to say some more numbers, but when I am through you must repeat them to me in the <u>backwards</u> order."* Read the three number sequence at a rate of one digit per second.

<u>Scoring</u>: Allocate one point for each sequence correctly repeated, (*N.B.*: the correct response for the backwards trial is 2-4-7).

<u>Vigilance: Administration</u>: The examiner reads the list of letters at a rate of one per second, after giving the following instruction: *"I am going to read a sequence of letters. Every time I say the letter A, tap your hand once. If I say a different letter, do not tap your hand"*.

<u>Scoring</u>: Give one point if there is zero to one errors (an error is a tap on a wrong letter or a failure to tap on letter A).

2

Table 2.2 Montreal Cognitive Assessment Tool (*Continued*)

Serial 7s: Administration: The examiner gives the following instruction: *"Now, I will ask you to count by subtracting seven from 100, and then, keep subtracting seven from your answer until I tell you to stop."* Give this instruction twice if necessary.

Scoring: This item is scored out of 3 points. Give no (0) points for no correct subtractions, 1 point for one correction subtraction, 2 points for two-to-three correct subtractions, and 3 points if the participant successfully makes four or five correct subtractions. Count each correct subtraction of 7 beginning at 100. Each subtraction is evaluated independently; that is, if the participant responds with an incorrect number but continues to correctly subtract 7 from it, give a point for each correct subtraction. For example, a participant may respond "92 – 85 – 78 – 71 – 64" where the "92" is incorrect, but all subsequent numbers are subtracted correctly. This is one error and the item would be given a score of 3.

7. **Sentence repetition:**

Administration: The examiner gives the following instructions: *"I am going to read you a sentence. Repeat it after me, exactly as I say it* [pause]: ***I only know that John is the one to help today."*** Following the response, say: *"Now I am going to read you another sentence. Repeat it after me, exactly as I say it* [pause]: ***The cat always hid under the couch when dogs were in the room."***

Scoring: Allocate 1 point for each sentence correctly repeated. Repetition must be exact. Be alert for errors that are omissions (e.g., omitting "only", "always") and substitutions/additions (e.g., "John is the one who helped today;" substituting "hides" for "hid", altering plurals, etc.).

8. **Verbal fluency:**

Administration: The examiner gives the following instruction: *"Tell me as many words as you can think of that begin with a certain letter of the alphabet that I will tell you in a moment. You can say any kind of word you want, except for proper nouns (like Bob or Boston), numbers, or words that begin with the same sound but have a different suffix, for example, love, lover, loving. I will tell you to stop after one minute. Are you ready?* [Pause] *Now, tell me as many words as you can think of that begin with the letter F.* [time for 60 sec]. *Stop."*

Scoring: Allocate one point if the subject generates 11 words or more in 60 sec. Record the subject's response in the bottom or side margins.

9. **Abstraction:**

Administration: The examiner asks the subject to explain what each pair of words has in common, starting with the example: *"Tell me how an orange and a banana are alike".* If the subject answers in a concrete manner, then say only one additional time: *"Tell me another way in which those items are alike".* If the subject does not give the appropriate response *(fruit)*, say, *"Yes, and they are also both fruit."* Do not give any additional instructions or clarification.
After the practice trial, say: *"Now, tell me how a train and a bicycle are alike".* Following the response, administer the second trial, saying: *"Now tell me how a ruler and a watch are alike".* Do not give any additional instructions or prompts.

Table 2.2   *(Continued)*

Scoring: Only the last two item pairs are scored. Give 1 point to each item pair correctly answered. The following responses are acceptable:

Train-bicycle = means of transportation, means of travelling, you take trips in both; Ruler-watch = measuring instruments, used to measure.

The following responses are **not** acceptable: Train-bicycle = they have wheels; Ruler-watch = they have numbers.

10.   Delayed recall:

Administration: The examiner gives the following instruction: "*I read some words to you earlier, which I asked you to remember. Tell me as many of those words as you can remember.* Make a check mark ($\checkmark$) for each of the words correctly recalled spontaneously without any cues, in the allocated space.

Scoring: **Allocate 1 point for each word recalled freely without any cues.**

> **Optional:**
> Following the delayed free recall trial, prompt the subject with the semantic category cue provided below for any word not recalled. Make a check mark ($\checkmark$) in the allocated space if the subject remembered the word with the help of a category or multiple-choice cue. Prompt all non-recalled words in this manner. If the subject does not recall the word after the category cue, give him/her a multiple choice trial, using the following example instruction, "*Which of the following words do you think it was, NOSE, FACE, or HAND?*"
> Use the following category and/or multiple-choice cues for each word, when appropriate:
> FACE: category cue: part of the body   multiple choice: nose, face, hand
> VELVET: category cue: type of fabric   multiple choice: denim, cotton, velvet
> CHURCH: category cue: type of building   multiple choice: church, school, hospital
> DAISY: category cue: type of flower   multiple choice: rose, daisy, tulip
> RED: category cue: a colour   multiple choice: red, blue, green
> Scoring: **No points are allocated for words recalled with a cue.** A cue is used for clinical information purposes only and can give the test interpreter additional information about the type of memory disorder. For memory deficits due to retrieval failures, performance can be improved with a cue. For memory deficits due to encoding failures, performance does not improve with a cue.

11.   Orientation:

Administration: The examiner gives the following instructions: "*Tell me the date today*". If the subject does not give a complete answer, then prompt accordingly by saying: "*Tell me the [year, month, exact date, and day of the week].*" Then say: "*Now, tell me the name of this place, and which city it is in.*"

Scoring: Give one point for each item correctly answered. The subject must tell the exact date and the exact place (name of hospital, clinic, office). No points are allocated if subject makes an error of one day for the day and date.

TOTAL SCORE: Sum all subscores listed on the right-hand side. Add one point for an individual who has 12 years or fewer of formal education, for a possible maximum of 30 points. A final total score of 26 and above is considered normal.

4

MoCA Version November 12, 2004
© *Z. Nasreddine MD*

                                                                                    www.mocatest.org

Source: Courtesy of Z. Nasreddine. Available at: http://www.mocatest.org.

- For *III, IV, and VI*, examine extraocular movements *up* (superior rectus), *down* (inferior rectus), *patient's right side* (lateral rectus on right, medial rectus on left), *left* (lateral rectus on left, medial rectus on right), upper right (inferior oblique on left, superior and lateral rectus on right), upper left (inferior oblique on right, superior and lateral rectus on left), lower right (superior oblique on left, inferior and lateral rectus on right), and lower left (superior oblique on right, inferior and lateral rectus on left).
- For *V*, check facial sensation to light touch and pinprick [all three divisions—forehead (V1), cheek (V2), lower mandible (V3)]; note that vibration testing for a unilateral deficit on the face or forehead is unreliable because the vibration easily travels along the bony skull. Check the muscles of mastication by opening and closing the jaw.
- For *VII*, check facial movement to eye closure and brow furrowing, showing teeth (or dentures), smiling. It is important to check the upper (brow, eyelids) and lower (nasolabial fold with smiling, or showing teeth) face.
- For *VIII*, check for hearing loss. Note: first check the external ear canal for wax. Ask the patient to repeat whispers given in front of patient while making masking noises (e.g., rubbing fingers) in front of the opposite ear. An alternative is to find the distance the patient can hear a ticking watch while making masking noises in the contralateral ear. Rinne and Webber tests are additional bedside tests to localize hearing loss (16,17).
- For *IX and X*, check the movement of palate (ahhhhhh), test gag reflex on each side at the tonsillar pillar area. Listen to the voice for hoarseness (recurrent laryngeal nerve).
- For *XI*, ask the patient to raise their shoulders (test trapezius strength), turn their head and hold [sternocleidomastoids (SCMs)—check that they contract]. Note that turning the head to the left tests the right SCM and turning the head to the right tests the left SCM. Neck flexion can also be examined.
- For *XII*, check if the protruded tongue is midline and appears normal (does not deviate, is not wasted). It is easy to be fooled by apparent tongue deviation; check tongue strength when it is pushed into the inside of the cheek. Check for tongue fasciculations without the tongue protruded. Definite fasciculations should not be confused with normal tongue muscle contractions from positioning.

Motor

The motor examination checks for bulk, power, tone, and coordination. A good screening test is to have the patient put his/her arms in front with eyes closed. With palms up, this tests for subtle corticospinal tract dysfunction (pronator drift). With palms down and wrists extended, this tests for tremor, asterixis or upward drift (proprioceptive deficit). Places to check for bulk (wasting) include intrinsic hand muscles, forearms, shoulder muscles (deltoid, supraspinatus, infraspinatus), quadriceps, anterior compartment lower limb muscles, gastrocnemius/soleus, and extensor digitorum brevis. Examples of muscles to quickly test/screen for weakness: deltoids, biceps, triceps, finger extensors, interossei, thumb abductors, hip flexors, quadriceps, hamstring, foot and toe dorsiflexion, foot plantar flexion. If weakness in a limb or nerve territory is suspected, more muscles can be added. In general, assess at least a proximal and distal upper and lower limb muscle. Examining extensor muscles (triceps, wrist extension, finger extension) and foot dorsiflexion checks for a "pyramidal" distribution of weakness seen in upper motor neuron damage.

To quickly check for coordination, use the finger-nose-finger (FNF) test and heel-shin (HS) test. Added tests include fine finger movements, for example, "touch each finger to your thumb as quickly and accurately as possible," or "tap your thumb with your index finger as rapidly as possible" (patients are often slightly faster and stronger on the dominant side), or toe tapping, especially if the patient is obese and unable to cooperate with the HS test.

Reflexes

Use a proper reflex hammer such as the Queen square model; the tomahawk hammer is too short and hard. Routinely check biceps, triceps, brachioradialis, quadriceps (knee), and ankle deep tendon reflexes. Always observe the muscle for contraction (make sure the relevant muscle is visible). The plantar responses are tested with a blunt probe. Begin with a gentle touch (this is not a test of pain sensation) and scraping or other vigorous stimuli can cause injury in diabetics with skin disease. The plantar response should be consistent with repeated testing.

Sensation

Check for sensory loss to light touch (cotton, brush), pinprick (clean safety pin— do *not* use a blood draw needle and do *not* reuse needles), thermal sensation [such as a cooled (e.g., held under cold water) tuning fork], vibration (128 Hz), and position sensation. Begin with the large toe. Establish if there is anesthesia (inability to feel any light touch) or analgesia (unable to distinguish sharp from dull) and then work proximally mapping any sensory deficit (to screen for polyneuropathy) and check each volar finger [to look for carpal tunnel syndrome (CTS), ulnar neuropathy]. Go from abnormal to normal with the patient's eyes closed, asking when the sensation has returned to normal. Also test for cortical sensory neglect by lightly touching both sides of the arms or legs, with the patient's eyes closed, and asking her/him to identify the side touched (known as double simultaneous stimulation). In cortical neglect, the patient routinely ignores sensation on one side when tested this way, while recognizing sensation on that side when it is tested alone. In general, sensory testing should include modalities served by large myelinated nerve fibers (light touch, vibration sense, joint position sense) and by small unmyelinated axons (pain, temperature) that travel in different parts of the nervous system. Consider adding a monofilament test (see the following text) to the routine examination.

Gait and Stance

Check normal walking, tandem walk [one foot in front of the next (may be difficult for very obese or pregnant patients)], and standing on toes/heels. To check for a Romberg sign, have the patient close their eyes, put their feet together (as long as this can be done with their eyes open without losing their stance), and the arms outstretched. A Romberg sign is a loss of stance, and the examiner must be prepared to steady the patient. Patients with foot ulcers may be unable to perform these tests.

Screening Neurological Examinations

- May be performed during brief visits in busy diabetes clinics
- Not indicated if a new and significant neurological problem has developed
- May be varied depending on screening requirements

Polyneuropathy Examination

- Examine distal sensation to light touch, pinprick, thermal sensation, and vibration [with patient eyes closed check for anesthesia (any sensation to touch?) and analgesia (can distinguish sharp and dull ends of a safety pin?)] in the foot (start from toe, work up) and hands (from volar fingers, work up)
- Test ankle and knee reflexes
- Test distal toe and foot dorsiflexion weakness
- Include Semmes–Weinstein monofilament test

Autonomic Neuropathy Examination

- Check BP and pulse lying, then again after standing for 60 seconds (after 1 minute; normal <20 mmHg systolic drop).
- Check pupillary reactions.
- Look for evidence of normal hand/foot sweating (dry feet, moist socks, etc.).

Carpal Tunnel Syndrome (CTS) Examination

- Look for thenar muscle wasting.
- Check light touch and pinprick in all of the fingers by beginning with the tips and working proximally until the sensation is normal; may be normal or abnormal in the distal fingers only, or in the whole median nerve sensory territory; sensation should normalize at the wrist and in the proximal thenar skin just distal to the wrist crease (the skin supplied by a sensory branch, the palmar cutaneous branch, that is spared in CTS).
- Check for a Tinel's sign—this is elicited by tapping at the wrist and is positive if it reproduces the tingling the patient experiences in the hand and fingers.

- Check for weakness of the abductor policis brevis (median nerve muscle) that raises the thumb vertically from the palm when the palm is faceup.
- Check for weakness of the biceps muscle (C5, C6 myotome and musculocutaneous nerve but not innervated by the median nerve) that should be normal in isolated CTS.

Ulnar Neuropathy at the Elbow (UNE) Examination

- Look for first dorsal interosseous (first web space) and hypothenar muscle wasting.
- Check for weakness of interosseous muscles (abduction and adduction) with preserved thenar (median) muscle power.
- Check for weakness of the flexor pollicis longus, which flexes the distal thumb. It is innervated by the C8 myotome and the anterior interosseus nerve; it should be normal in cases of UNE.
- Check light touch and pinprick in all of the fingers by beginning with the tips and working proximally until the sensation is normal; may be normal, or more often loss of sensation involves the small and medial half of the ring finger; ringer finger splitting is helpful for the diagnosis; sensory loss should not extend up the forearm.
- Check if sensory symptoms can be reproduced by rolling the ulnar nerve in the cubital tunnel at the elbow.
- Check if the elbow ulnar groove is abnormally shallow or if the carrying angle of the arm is abnormal (inability to fully extend the elbow predisposes patients to UNE).

Is There Subtle Hemiparesis?

- Observe facial movement (check nasolabial fold).
- Check for pronator drift of the outstretched hand.
- Check for reflex asymmetry and an upgoing plantar response on the hemiparetic side.
- Determine the presence of abnormal gait instability, that is, the patient may circumduct the involved side.
- If any abnormalities are identified, a comprehensive neurological examination is required.

Dementia Assessment

MoCA (Table 2.2)
See chapter 3

Neuropathy Scales

See chapter 9

NEUROLOGICAL INVESTIGATIONS

Nerve Conduction Studies and Electromyography

- Performed by neurologists and physiatrists.
- An extension of the neurological examination.
- Procedure is sometimes referred to as "EMG studies."
- Requires special training and certification [e.g., American Board of Electro-diagnostic Medicine (ABEM) in the United States, Canadian Society of Clinical Neurophysiologists (CSCN) in Canada].
- Nerve conduction can be performed by certified technologists under direct supervision, but needle electromyography (EMG) is carried out by a physician.
- Does not require anesthesia or analgesia; there is minor and transient discomfort [electrical stimuli for nerve conduction, electrode (needle) insertion into muscles for EMG].
- Disposable needles have largely replaced sterilized, reusable needles.
- EMG (but not nerve conduction) is relatively contraindicated in anti-coagulated patients (risk of hematoma), those with low platelets (<50,000/microliter) or patients with bleeding disorders.
- A report should detail motor conduction velocity, sensory conduction velocity, median nerve distal motor latency (DMLs), and amplitudes of the motor and sensory responses (CMAPs and SNAPs, see definition in the following text). The studies should routinely include both sides with limb temperature documented. Diabetic polyneuropathy causes slowing of conduction velocities and loss of motor and sensory potentials beginning in the feet (Table 2.3).

Technical Primer

Nerve conduction studies are performed in hospitals or clinics to diagnose and evaluate the type, severity, and course of neuropathies. They are often combined with EMG studies at the same setting but the EMG component is not always required.

Nerve conduction studies involve brief (0.1–0.5 msec in duration) electrical stimuli applied over landmarks on the skin that identify nerve trunks close to the surface. The technique involves stimulation on the surface of the skin over the nerve trunk at one or more sites along the course of the nerve. Stimulation is titrated to excite all of the myelinated axons of the nerve trunk.

CMAPS are compound muscle action potentials recorded from the muscle endplate. To generate a CMAP, action potentials travel down motor axons, cross the neuromuscular junction at the endplate, and then excite the muscle membrane. The amplitude (size) of the CMAP therefore reflects (*i*) the number of intact or excitable motor axons; (*ii*) the state of neuromuscular junction transmission; and (*iii*) the number of excitable muscle fibers. The distal motor latency (DML) is the time for the CMAP to appear when stimulating at the most distal site, close to the muscle; in the case of the median nerve, the time for the

Table 2.3 Summary of Neurological Tests for Diabetic Patients

Test	Role
Nerve conduction and EMG	To gauge severity of neuropathy
	To follow patients if specific treatment prescribed
	To rule out other types of neuropathy where possible
	Not required as a screening test
Nerve biopsy	*Not* a routine test; use for specific indications only
Semmes–Weinstein monofilament	Screening for polyneuropathy together with an abbreviated neurological exam
Graduated tuning fork	Screening for polyneuropathy together with an abbreviated neurological exam
Computerized QST	Adjunct for following patients, not for screening
Skin biopsy	Role uncertain beyond research protocols
Corneal confocal microscopy	Role uncertain beyond research protocols but shows promise as a painless, rapid diagnostic tool
Autonomic testing	For patients with prominent autonomic complaints
Imaging	For CNS indications including stroke (cerebral infarction or hemorrhage), TIA, suspected spinal cord disease or disc protrusions, other; to exclude plexus tumors or infiltration

Abbreviations: EMG, electromyography; QST, quantitative sensory testing; CNS, central nervous system; TIA, transient ischemic attack.

stimulation to travel from the wrist through the carpal tunnel and to the muscle endplate in the hand (thenar abductor pollicis brevis muscle). DMLs of the median nerve are prolonged in CTS. Conduction velocities are calculated in more proximal segments of the nerve (e.g., forearm, across the elbow, leg from knee to ankle). If the nerve is stimulated distally (e.g., median nerve at the wrist) or proximally (e.g., median nerve at the elbow), CMAPs should be about the same size. If there is a 30% to 50% fall in the amplitude (or area) of the proximal response without a significant widening of the CMAP, the change is referred to as conduction block. Conduction block implies that there is demyelination between the distal and proximal stimulating site; this is less common in diabetic polyneuropathy. Similarly, the CMAP may become spread out, or dispersed along the course of the nerve, a further feature of demyelination. F waves are smaller waves that are recorded in the tracing after the CMAP. They are from motor potentials that travel to the spinal cord, then return to the motor endplate (long loop reflexes). They can have a prolonged latency time in polyneuropathy.

SNAPs are compound *sensory nerve action potentials* that arise from all of the large myelinated axons in the nerve trunk beneath the recording electrode. Nerve conduction studies do not routinely assess small unmyelinated axons or autonomic axons. The amplitude of the SNAP reflects the number of intact or excitable sensory axons and how well synchronized they travel (the SNAP

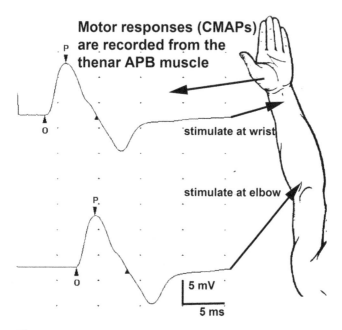

Figure 2.1 Nerve conduction study of the median motor nerve. This test is used to identify CTS. The site, over the abductor pollicus brevis muscle, where the motor response (CMAP) is recorded is indicated. The median nerve is stimulated at the wrist and at the elbow. *Abbreviations*: CTS, carpal tunnel syndrome; CMAP, compound muscle action potential; APB, abductor pollicis brevis.

represents the summation of all of the individual action potentials of each axon from hundreds found in the nerve trunk); if a significant number are inordinately slowed or not synchronized, they do not summate well and the SNAP is smaller in amplitude.

Commonly tested nerves and their stimulation sites are as follows:

Median nerve motor conduction recording over the abductor pollicus brevis in the thenar eminence (2-point stimulation: wrist and elbow). Median sensory conduction recording over the index finger (1- or 2-point stimulation: wrist and elbow) (Figs. 2.1 and 2.2).

Ulnar nerve motor conduction recording over the abductor digiti minimi in the hypothenar eminence (3-point stimulation: wrist, below elbow, and above elbow). Ulnar sensory conduction recording over the fifth (small) digit (1- or 3-point stimulation: wrist, below elbow, and above elbow). The ulnar nerve may also be stimulated in the axilla or at Erb's point above the clavicle.

Radial nerve sensory conduction recording over the nerve at the base of the thumb (1-point stimulation: distal forearm).

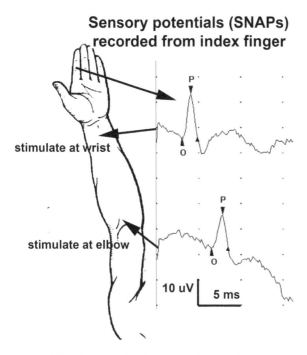

Figure 2.2 Nerve conduction study of the median sensory nerve. This study is also used to identify CTS. The site, over the index finger digital nerves, where the sensory response (SNAP) is recorded is indicated. The median nerve is stimulated at the wrist and at the elbow. This type of sensory conduction is termed "antidromic" since the nerve is stimulated proximally and recorded distally (reverse direction of normal sensation). *Abbreviations*: CTS, carpal tunnel syndrome; SNAP, sensory nerve action potential.

Peroneal nerve motor conduction recording over the extensor digitorum brevis on the dorsum of the foot (3-point stimulation: ankle, fibular head, knee). Peroneal nerve sensory conduction recording over the nerve on the dorsum of the ankle (1-point stimulation: lower leg).
Tibial nerve motor conduction recording over abductor hallucis in the instep of the foot (2-point stimulation: ankle, knee).
Sural nerve sensory conduction recording over the nerve below the lateral malleolus (1-point stimulation: distal calf) (Fig. 2.3).

Most studies focus on one side of the body: one arm and leg are examined for the presence of a presumed symmetrical polyneuropathy. If there is an abnormality on one side of the patient, the contralateral side should then be checked (or routinely done for upper limb problems, see the following text). All four limbs are studied in more complex cases. The most sensitive nerves for diabetic

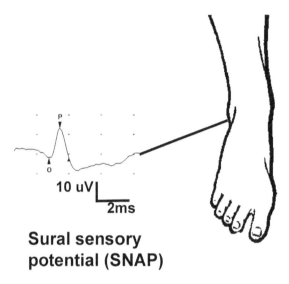

**Sural sensory
potential (SNAP)**

Figure 2.3 Nerve conduction study of the sural sensory nerve. Sural sensory nerve conduction is the most sensitive electrophysiological index of diabetic polyneuropathy. The diagram points to the site, behind the ankle, where the sensory nerve action potential (SNAP) is recorded. The nerve is stimulated over the posterior calf.

polyneuropathy are sural sensory conduction studies and peroneal motor conduction. Median studies (bilateral recommended) are essential for the diagnosis of CTS and ulnar nerve studies (also bilateral recommended) for ulnar neuropathy at the elbow (UNE).

EMG is carried out at the same sitting as nerve conduction but may not always be required. It involves the insertion of fine sterile, disposable recording needles into muscle. Two main pieces of information are evaluated. First, the muscle is recorded at rest. Abnormal spontaneous activity, known as fibrillations or positive sharp waves, is identified when the muscle fibers are denervated (loss of its nerve supply). The density of abnormal spontaneous activity (numbers of fibrillations, positive sharp waves) and its distribution (e.g., in median innervated muscles in the hand in severe CTS but not in adjacent ulnar innervated muscles) indicate the severity and the pattern of denervation. Muscle inflammation (e.g., polymyositis) can also cause abnormal spontaneous activity. Secondly, the patient voluntarily activates the muscle. The number, size, and shape of the recruited motor units may be helpful (e.g., they are enlarged in chronic partial denervated muscles but reduced in size in muscle disorders).

There are additional but less routine electrophysiological studies: blink reflexes (for facial numbness or paralysis), repetitive conduction studies (for myasthenia gravis), motor unit estimates, somatosensory evoked potentials, sympathetic skin potentials (SSR), single fiber EMG (SFEMG for myasthenia gravis), and other less common nerve territory conduction recordings not reviewed here.

Caveats About Nerve Conduction and EMG

- Interpretations and results can be incorrect and substantially misleading if not performed in a qualified, certified laboratory.
- Good quality results are highly reproducible and are among the most sensitive indices of diabetic polyneuropathy.
- The report should include clinical history, examination, numbers (distal latencies, conduction velocities, amplitudes) for each nerve, preferably the waveforms also, and an interpretation of the results.
- Extremities (especially hands) should be warmed prior to testing (at least 32°C for the hand, 30°C for the foot). The temperature should be documented.
- Sensory conduction velocities reflect those of the fastest myelinated axons; they do not provide information about unmyelinated axons (e.g., those transmitting pain) and do not strictly correlate with neurological symptoms.
- EMG needle recordings may not be abnormal immediately after a nerve injury. Fibrillations take one to two weeks to appear in denervated muscle fibers.
- Nerve conduction may be normal in mild peripheral neuropathies, including mild diabetic polyneuropathy.

When Are Nerve Conduction and EMG Testing Required?

- To determine whether a polyneuropathy can be attributed to diabetes mellitus (may rule out other types of polyneuropathy)
- For the diagnosis of polyneuropathy in some patients when the cause of numbness or weakness is not clear. For example, completely normal studies in a patient with limb numbness or weakness may suggest a spinal cord disorder
- To follow the course of polyneuropathy in some patients
- To diagnose CTS, UNE, and other focal neuropathies that are common in diabetes

Nerve Biopsy

- Not routinely used in the diagnosis of diabetic peripheral neuropathy.
- Used in the diagnosis of progressive and significant neuropathy in which a diagnosis other than diabetes mellitus is being considered: for example, amyloidosis, vasculitis, chronic inflammatory demyelinating polyneuropathy (CIDP).

- The sural nerve usually chosen if a biopsy is required and a whole nerve rather than fascicular biopsy is preferred. The sural nerve supplies the lateral side of the foot and ankle. The patient should have clinical sensory loss in the distribution of the sural nerve and an abnormal SNAP before a sural nerve biopsy is considered.
- Careful patient consent is required for this invasive procedure; there is a risk of infection in diabetics or ulcer formation in patients with significant vascular disease.
- A sural nerve biopsy leaves an area of sensory loss and can cause mild neuropathic pain (generally rated as mild, graded as 2–3/10 and slowly resolving) in its territory (18).

Quantitative Sensory Testing

Simple Devices

1. Semmes–Weinstein 10 g monofilament test. The monofilament is pressed against the dorsum of the large toe (plantar application has also been described) until it bends and the patient (with eyes closed) is asked to identify when the stimuli are applied. For example, one may score the number of times the monofilament is felt out of five trials on the top of each toe.
2. Rydel Seiffer 64/128 Hz graduated tuning fork. This is a special tuning fork with adjustable dampers screwed into the arms of each shaft. When the dampers are off, the fork vibrates at 128 Hz. When they are on and tightened at the appropriate place on the shaft, they vibrate at 64 Hz. When the patient stops sensing vibration, a numerical readout is visible from images of intersecting triangles on each damper.

Computerized Systems

- An adjunct to clinical examination, not a screening method or approach.
- Originally developed by Dyck and colleagues at Mayo Clinic, but now several commercial varieties are marketed (Mayo Clinic setup marketed as CASE IV—Computerized Assisted Sensory Examination IV).
- Capable of testing several modalities of sensation.
- Careful quiet nondistracted testing conditions are required; the most reliable approaches involve a forced-choice paradigm.
- All results require comparison to age and gender-matched controls.
- Useful for longitudinal follow-up of patients.
- Be cautious about nonvalidated setups (e.g., portable hand held setups) and devices that detect nonphysiological stimuli (e.g., current perception).
- Modalities tested for by quantitative sensory testing (QST) include vibration perception threshold (VPT; likely the most commonly used form of QST in clinical trials) but also touch-pressure, warm and cool detection

thresholds (WDT and CDT), and heat as pain (HNDT, or heat-nociception detection threshold). CASE IV can be used for VPT, WDT, CDT, and HNDT (19). QST abnormalities in clinical trials correlate with other measures of diabetic polyneuropathy (20).

Skin Biopsy

- A new approach toward the diagnosis of loss of small fibers (axons) in early polyneuropathy
- Uses local anesthesia and involves a 3-mm punch biopsy through the epidermis and into the dermis and subdermis
- Less invasive than a nerve biopsy
- Requires a specialized lab that can perform immunohistochemistry of axons (labeled with an antibody to PGP 9.5, a molecule that is expressed in all axons) and that can reproducibly provide quantitative fiber counts
- Relatively few laboratories worldwide carry out this procedure, but it is slowly gaining acceptance
- Distal sites, such as the dorsum of foot, are the most sensitive places to detect abnormalities
- Caution is advised in diabetic patients with poor foot care, ulcers, or poor glucose control (risk of infection)

Punch biopsies of the skin are used to examine epidermal skin innervation by small axons as a sensitive index of neuropathy. Standardized approaches toward the sampling and processing of skin biopsies and the measurement of the linear density of intraepidermal skin fibers (IENF) have been proposed by the European Federation of Neurological Societies (21). Diabetic polyneuropathy is associated with a reduction in the density of IENF and other changes such as the presence of degenerative axonal ovoid structures.

Corneal Confocal Microscopy

- A new noninvasive way to assess neuropathy by analyzing the nerve fibers in the cornea with a clinical microscope
- Requires patient cooperation but is otherwise simple and rapid; methodology for counting the fibers needs to be standardized
- Recently identified as a sensitive and noninvasive approach toward assessing diabetic polyneuropathy, corneal confocal microscopy (CCM) examines corneal innervation using microscopy to scan the cornea for the nerve plexus of Bowman's layer. Malik and colleagues initially described the technique in 18 diabetic patients and 18 age-matched control subjects and identified reductions in fiber density, length, and branch density in diabetic patients, particularly those with severe diabetic polyneuropathy (22)

Autonomic Nervous System Testing

- A series of tests to evaluate different parts of the autonomic nervous system (see chap. 13):
- Forms of testing include (*i*) evaluation of cardiovascular autonomic neuropathy (RR interval variation at rest, with deep breathing, with Valsalva maneuver; blood pressure response to standing, Valsalva or isometric exercise; spectral analysis); (*ii*) nocturnal penile tumescence and rigidity for erectile dysfunction; (*iii*) gastrointestinal motility and manometry tests for gastrointestinal neuropathy; (*iv*) cystometrogram for bladder function; and (*v*) evaluation of sweating (QSART, quantitative sudomotor axon reflex testing; TST, thermoregulatory sweat test) (23).

Magnetic Resonance and Other Forms of Imaging

- Useful for assessing the brain, spinal cord, nerve roots, plexus, and muscles
- Not helpful in the diagnosis of peripheral polyneuropathy or entrapment neuropathy
- For cerebral infarction (stroke), consider brain MR with MR angiography and include diffusion imaging to assess recent ischemic damage
- For urgent evaluation of cerebral vessels, including the carotid bifurcation, consider CT angiography of the brain and neck vessels but use with caution in diabetics because of potential renal damage from CT contrast

3

Neurological presentations

In this chapter, we describe a number of neurological problems as they present to the health care provider. Brief guidelines are presented for their diagnosis and management.

ACUTE CONFUSION IN A DIABETIC PATIENT

KEY POINTS

- Identify whether there is hypoglycemia first.
- Evaluate for hypotension, cardiac arrhythmia.
- Is it confusion or aphasia? Aphasia is a focal deficit in speech comprehension or output.
- Is there evidence of infection?
- Is there visual loss? Bilateral visual loss can cause apparent confusion.
- Was there a recent seizure?

Is There a Metabolic Reason for Confusion?

- Hypoglycemia—may be preceded by anxiety, sweating, tachycardia; history of insulin use with reduced calorie intake or excessive exercise
- Hyperglycemia—diabetic ketoacidosis, nonketotic hyperosmolar syndrome
- Severe hypothyroidism with decompensation ("myxedema madness")
- Other

Is There Hypotension?

- Causes may include postural hypotension, myocardial infarction, GI bleed, pulmonary embolism, septic shock

Is Aphasia Mistaken for Confusion?

- Receptive aphasia may have nonsensical speech, word or letter substitutions. Patient is fluent but speech cannot be interpreted. The patient cannot repeat or follow commands.
- Patients with motor aphasia may have limited, one- or two-word phrases without meaningful speech, and they cannot repeat but can follow commands. Patients are often frustrated and may be agitated.

Is It Drug or Analgesia Induced?

- Patients may have an underlying pain problem (neuropathy, other) and have escalated their intake of analgesics.
- Polypharmacy (especially multiple analgesics with or without sedatives) is a risk factor for confusion.
- Associated abdominal pain, constipation, small pupils, and confusion may suggest opioid overuse.
- This is a more common problem in older patients with other medical problems.

Was There a Recent Head Injury?

- Check for signs of trauma, Battle's sign (defined as ecchymosis behind the ear secondary to a basal skull fracture), hemotympanum, other injuries (e.g., rib fractures).
- Ataxia, frontal lobe release signs, and confusion may suggest unilateral or bilateral subdural hematomas.

Is There an Infection?

- Signs of neurological infection may be masked in diabetes (fever, stiff neck).
- Suspect meningitis in subacute-acute confusion without focal signs and normal imaging.
- Diabetic persons have an increased risk of unusual infections (see chap. 15).
- Suspect herpes simplex encephalitis (HSE) with acute confusion, fever, speech difficulties, progressive worsening; CT brain scan often normal in early HSE.
- Older patients with preexisting neurological impairment (multiple cerebral infarcts, dementia) may develop confusion in the setting of a systemic infection such as a urinary tract infection, pneumonia, sepsis.
- Signs of an acute abdomen may not be present in a diabetic person (appendicitis, diverticulitis, cholecystitis, other).

Was There a Recent Stroke?

- Suggested by a previous history of stroke (cerebral infarction or hemorrhage), TIA, coronary artery disease, peripheral vascular disease.

- Suggested by the presence of risk factors for cerebrovascular disease.
- Cerebrovascular disease is suspected when a carotid bruit from internal carotid artery stenosis is identified.
- Associated neurological signs and symptoms—weakness, ataxia, upgoing toe(s), unilateral hyperreflexia, neglect, visual field defect may indicate a prior stroke.
- Acute confusion may complicate unilateral or bifrontal cerebral infarcts or nondominant parietal infarcts.
- Brain imaging, in particular diffusion weighted brain MR, may be required to determine if there is an area of acute ischemia or hemorrhage.

Other Causes

- Bilateral visual or hearing loss in an older person.
- Patients with a preexisting mild cognitive disorder may decompensate in hospital from a loss of normal surroundings and an added medical disorder, a syndrome termed "beclouded dementia."
- If there is agitated confusion in a patient already in hospital for two to three days consider delirium tremens from ethanol withdrawal.
- Nonconvulsive status epilepticus (NCSE) may be associated with a prolonged confusional state: clues may be fluctuating level of consciousness, upgoing plantar responses, automatisms (blinking, repetitive hand movements), and a history of cerebral disease or seizures.

Differential Diagnosis

- Metabolic-hypoglycemia, hyperglycemia, hyponatremia, hypernatremia, hypocalcemia, hypercalcemia
- Nondominant parietal or bilateral stroke (cerebral infarction or hemorrhage)
- Drug intoxication (prescription or street drugs)
- Ethanol or drug withdrawal
- Head injury
- NCSE
- Postictal confusion (following a seizure)
- CNS infection—early encephalitis, meningitis
- Transient global amnesia

FOCAL WEAKNESS IN A DIABETIC PATIENT

KEY POINTS

- It is critical to localize the type of weakness: peripheral nervous system (PNS) involving one or more nerve territories and central nervous system (CNS).
- Unilateral arm and leg weakness are less likely to be from neuropathy.
- Upper motor neuron signs may be masked in diabetes (see chap. 4).
- Imaging studies are helpful to localize and characterize CNS lesions, and electrophysiology is useful to evaluate for PNS lesions.

Diagnosis

Localize the Lesion

1. One nerve, plexus, or nerve root territory
   - Upper limb—ulnar neuropathy (hand weakness, medial hand numbness; chronic), radial neuropathy (wrist drop with or without dorsal hand numbness; "acute"—patient may awaken with it), brachial neuritis (upper arm weakness, wasting and pain without sensory loss; subacute—over 1–2 days), radiculopathy (weakness, sensory loss, and radiating neck pain; may be acute-subacute).
   - Lower limb—peroneal neuropathy (foot drop, dorsal foot numbness; acute-subacute), lumbosacral plexopathy (thigh pain, weakness, and wasting; subacute), radiculopathy (weakness, sensory loss, and radiating back pain; may be acute-subacute).
2. Facial involvement
   - Suggests a cerebral lesion if it occurs in addition to limb weakness (motor cortex or internal capsule): lower facial weakness only, may be more apparent with smiling than nonemotional facial movement.
   - Peripheral facial weakness (Bell's palsy) involves all portions of the facial nerve with impaired forehead wrinkling, weakness of the lower face, and inability to fully close the eye.
3. Upper and lower limb involvement
   - Suggests a cerebral (motor cortex or internal capsule), brain stem, or upper spinal cord lesion.
   - Presence of a sensory level suggests a spinal cord lesion.
   - Contralateral loss of sensation to pinprick and temperature suggests a partial spinal cord lesion (Brown-Séquard syndrome).
   - Prominent loss of sphincter control suggests a spinal cord lesion.
   - Additional facial involvement suggests hemiparesis from cerebral lesion (above).
   - Additional cranial nerve abnormalities suggest a brain stem lesion: oculomotor (midbrain), abducens (pons), contralateral facial weakness, or facial numbness (medulla and pons).
   - Headache suggests an intracranial cause including migraine syndromes.
4. Reflexes
   - Brisk with upper motor neuron lesions (cortical, internal capsule, brain stem, spinal cord) but may be reduced in acute lesions.
   - Loss of a reflex in a weak muscle suggests a peripheral nerve, plexus, or nerve root lesion.
   - Upgoing plantar response suggests upper motor lesion, unless it is a confounding finding from an older lesion (e.g., old lacunar stroke).
   - Polyneuropathy, with reflex loss, may cloud neurological signs of an upper motor neuron lesion (see chap. 4).

5. Bilateral lower limbs
   - Suggest spinal cord problem, especially if there is a sensory level, brisk reflexes in weak muscles, loss of abdominal reflexes, upgoing toes, bowel and bladder involvement.
   - Occasional cases of diabetic lumbosacral plexopathy (DLSP) exhibit bilateral lower limb weakness, although involvement of one leg usually follows that of the other by several weeks.

What is the Type of Lesion?

1. Acute onset
   - Without provocation suggests cerebral ischemia or hemorrhage (hemiparesis from cerebral infarct or hemorrhage, ischemic oculomotor palsy)
   - On awakening suggests cerebral infarction, some compression palsies (e.g., radial neuropathy), or symptomatic carpal tunnel syndrome
   - With activity (e.g., lifting or twisting) suggests a radiculopathy
2. Subacute onset
   - Causes include DLSP, weakness secondary to a growing mass lesion (cerebral primary or secondary tumors, intraspinal tumors, plexus tumors, nerve tumors), or weakness secondary to an inflammatory lesion [sarcoidosis, multiple sclerosis (MS), other]
3. Chronic
   - Causes include entrapment neuropathy, radiculopathy, plexopathy, inflammatory lesions, or weakness from a slow-growing neoplasm

Associated Features

1. Prominent pain and focal weakness
   - Lumbosacral plexopathy (DLSP), radiculopathy, some entrapment neuropathies
2. Altered level of consciousness and focal weakness
   - Hypoglycemic hemiparesis, large intracranial lesion (infarction, hemorrhage, enlarging mass), hyperosmolar coma, hepatic encephalopathy, superimposed entrapment neuropathy in addition to a separate intracranial lesion, postictal deficit from a focally originating seizure that has become generalized
   - Post-traumatic—consider nerve or plexus damage (e.g., lumbosacral plexopathy from pelvic fracture), nerve root avulsion
   - Altered level of consciousness from ketoacidosis, hyperosmolar coma, hypoglycemia superimposed on a preexisting lesion

Investigations

- "Stat" glucose level in acute presentations
- Detailed neurological examination
- Tailor investigations according to the findings, clinical localization

- Brain CT, CTA (CT angiogram; see cautions on the use of CT contrast, chap. 4), brain MR (including diffusion weighting), and MRA (magnetic resonance angiography) for hemiparesis from cerebral lesions
- Spinal MR with gadolinium for hemiparesis or paraparesis from possible cord lesions
- Electrophysiological studies for peripheral nerve, plexus, and nerve root lesions

LEG PAIN IN A DIABETIC PATIENT

KEY POINTS

- Pain distribution is essential to determining the cause
- Identify whether the features of the pain suggest a neuropathic origin
- It is incorrect to assume that most types of lower limb pain are secondary to diabetes; it is essential to rule out other causes if the clinical features are atypical

History

What is the Distribution of the Pain?

- *Symmetrical distal*—polyneuropathy (e.g., mild in toes alone, moderate involving feet to ankles, severe involving the leg from feet to knees)
- *Unilateral*—radicular, in a nerve root territory (L3: thigh; L4: thigh, knee, below knee; L5: top of foot, lateral leg; S1: sole of foot, lateral side of foot; S2: posterior thigh, perianal). Most lumbar disks compress the root *below* the disk level, that is, L45 disk compresses L5, L5S1 disk compresses S1 (exceptions for this rule are far lateral disk protrusions that instead compress the root above), early mononeuritis multiplex, unilateral lumbosacral plexopathy, meralgia paresthetica (compression neuropathy of lateral femoral cutaneous nerve of the thigh)
- *Asymmetric bilateral*—mononeuritis multiplex (vasculitis, diabetes rarely, many other causes), bilateral radiculopathies (central disk—usually impairs bowel, bladder function; root infiltration by inflammation or tumor), spinal stenosis, bilateral lumbosacral plexopathy
- *Associated back pain, radiation*—root compression from disk, spinal stenosis

How is the Pain Described?

- *Burning, nocturnal, tender to touch (allodynia)*—polyneuropathy
- *Lancinating, electrical, sharp*—root (radiculopathy), mononeuritis multiplex, polyneuropathy
- *Deep boring and aching*—lumbosacral plexopathy
- *Combinations of the above*—polyneuropathy, radiculopathy, mononeuritis multiplex, plexopathy

Alleviating and Exacerbating Features

- *Better with sitting*—spinal stenosis
- *Worse with lying flat, standing, walking*—spinal stenosis
- *Worse at night, when resting*—polyneuropathy

Timing

- *Acute*—root compression from disk, mononeuritis multiplex, ischemia, deep venous thrombosis
- *Chronic*—polyneuropathy, spinal stenosis
- *Subacute (days to weeks)*—lumbosacral plexopathy, root compression, polyneuropathy exacerbation, bony lesion

Neurological Examination

- Color change, loss of pulses—ischemia
- Lesion on foot—infected ulcer
- Swelling, superficial venous engorgement, Homan's sign (calf pain with passive ankle dorsiflexion when the knee is flexed at 90°)—deep venous thrombosis (negative Homan's does not exclude deep venous thrombosis!)
- Swollen ankle—Charcot joint
- Red, warm, swollen base of large toe—acute gout
- Enlarged inguinal lymph nodes—tumor infiltration of plexus
- Flank hematoma—retroperitoneal hematoma with plexus compression
- Absent ankle reflexes—polyneuropathy
- Absent knee reflex—lumbosacral plexopathy or L34 disk
- Positive Lasègue's (straight leg raising)—root compression from disk
- Thigh wasting—lumbosacral plexopathy (or L34 disk)
- Sphincter tone abnormal, absent anal wink—central disk, cauda equina
- Unilateral upgoing toe or hyperreflexia with sphincter dysfunction—conus lesion
- Femoral stretch sign (pain on leg extension with patient lying on their side)—lumbosacral plexus damage from tumor, infiltration, inflammation

Investigations

- Rule out deep venous thrombosis (d-Dimer assay on blood, leg ultrasound)
- Rule out ischemia if suspected—urgent referral, may need MR angiography, ultrasound, or other arterial studies
- For suspected root disease—MR lumbar intraspinal space (add gadolinium enhancement if infiltrative problem suspected), possible CSF sampling (for suspected inflammation, tumor)
- For plexopathy—MR lumbar intraspinal space as above *plus* specific views of each lumbosacral plexus (with gadolinium); CT scan of pelvis, plexus may substitute for MR but should not replace the lumbar intraspinal MR study

- Radiographs or technetium isotope bone scan to identify a bony or bone marrow lesion
- Nerve conduction and electromyography are critical for investigation of a neuropathic cause

SEIZURES IN A DIABETIC PATIENT

KEY POINTS

- Assume patient is hypoglycemic and treat with 50% glucose intravenously.
- Follow glucose load with thiamine 100 mg intravenously.
- If the seizure is not secondary to hypoglycemia or hyperglycemia, manage it identically to a nondiabetic patient.
- Differing seizure types may have important implications: a focal seizure with or without secondary generalization may suggest a structural lesion of the cerebral cortex; a generalized tonic-clonic seizure may be secondary to primary generalized epilepsy or a metabolic abnormality.
- Patients with single seizures, a normal neurological examination and normal investigations may not require antiepileptic therapy.
- Status epilepticus (SE) is defined as greater than 30 minutes of continuous seizure activity or two or more sequential seizures without full recovery of consciousness
- Imaging studies are essential to identify whether there is an intracranial lesion causing seizures

Clinical Diagnosis

Evaluation of a Seizure Patient

- A detailed history is essential to identify predisposing factors: previous head injury, substance abuse, history of prior seizures, family history of seizures, history of febrile convulsion as an infant or a CNS infection; a history of febrile convulsions may lead to a diagnosis of mesial temporal sclerosis that is a pathological seizure focus for temporal lobe complex partial seizures.
- Details of other early life events and developmental history are helpful if available
- An aura preceding the seizure may help to localize its point of origin, for example, visual phenomena in seizures arising in the occipital lobe
- Information from an eyewitness is very helpful in identifying the circumstances of the seizure including premonitory behavior, duration, and other characteristics of the seizure
- Look for signs of unrecognized previous seizures: awakening with tongue or mouth bitten, sore muscles, or fractures

- Is there a history of recurrent hypoglycemia? This may suggest that there are ongoing occult hypoglycemia-related seizures
- Other diagnoses that resemble seizures: nonepileptic seizures (formerly called "psychogenic," no EEG correlate, no true loss of awareness, downgoing toes, forced "voluntary" eye closure, other clues), syncope with myoclonic movements (from hypotension), sleep behavior disorder, restless legs syndrome

Classification of the Seizure Type

A simple traditional classification: [see Table 3.1 for the updated International League Against Epilepsy (ILAE) full classification of seizures]:

- Focal (simple, partial) seizures—these are seizures arising from a single area of the cortex. Consciousness is retained. The symptoms may identify specific areas of involvement: sensory symptoms (paresthesiae, tingling, pain) from the parietal lobe, motor symptoms (muscle jerking) from the

Table 3.1 Summary of International League Against Epilepsy Updated (2010) Classification of Seizures

Generalized seizures	
Tonic-clonic (in any combination)	
Absence	Typical
	Atypical
	Absence with special features
	Myoclonic absence
	Eyelid myoclonia
Myoclonic	Myoclonic
	Myoclonic atonic
	Myoclonic tonic
Clonic	
Tonic	
Atonic	
Focal Seizures	
Without impairment of consciousness/responsiveness	
With impairment of consciousness/responsiveness (roughly corresponds to the concept of complex partial seizure)	
Evolving to a bilateral, convulsive seizure (involving tonic, clonic, or tonic and clonic components; replaces the term secondarily generalized seizure)	
May be focal, generalized, or unclear	
Epileptic spasms	

Source: Reproduced and summarized from www.ilae-epilepsy.org with permission. Please refer for full details to Berg AT, Berkovic SF, Brodie MJ, et al. Revised terminology and concepts for organization of seizures and epilepsies: Report of the ILAE Commission on Classification and Terminology, 2005–2009. Epilepsia 2010; 51:676–685.

motor cortex, visual symptoms (unformed or formed images) from the occipital or posterior temporal lobe, symptoms from the medial temporal or medial frontal lobes [rising sensations in abdomen and chest, olfactory and gustatory hallucinations, déjà vu (apparent familiarity when none should exist) and jamais vu (unfamiliarity when there should be familiarity), unwarranted fear], bilateral tonic posturing from the supplementary motor cortex in the frontal lobe, eye and head deviation away from a frontal lobe focus, nose rubbing by the hand ipsilateral to the seizure focus.

- Complex partial seizures (now called hippocampal or parahippocampal)—loss of awareness is the key feature either at outset of the seizure or later, after a focal seizure with temporal/frontal lobe symptoms that becomes a complex partial seizure; there may be automatisms (repetitive semipuposeful movements such as hand wringing, lip smacking).
- Secondary generalized seizures—begins as a focal seizure, then progresses to a generalized seizure with loss of consciousness and a tonic, clonic, or tonic-clonic seizure.
- Generalized onset—tonic, clonic, or tonic-clonic ("Grand mal" seizure) or absence seizures ("Petit mal" seizure). These occur with loss of awareness. Generalized onset tonic-clonic seizures often begin with vocalization, tonic arching with eyes rolled back, followed by bilateral synchronous clonic movements of the trunk and limbs, with frothing at the mouth, urinary and bowel incontinence, tongue and mouth biting. The patient may regain consciousness and note bleeding in the mouth, painful stiff muscles, incontinence, and occasionally injury with vertebral compression or rib fractures. Patients with generalized tonic, clonic, or tonic-clonic seizures usually have upgoing plantar responses during the seizure and for a few minutes after the seizure has ended. Generalized seizures are associated with an elevated body temperature, mild-moderate leukocytosis and neutrophilia, metabolic acidosis, transient hypoxia, elevated prolactin, and occasionally a few leukocytes in the CSF.

Localizing the Lesion

- Generalized seizures can occur from a diffuse abnormality of the cerebral cortex but may also arise from focal lesions.
- Complex partial seizures originate in the temporal or medial frontal lobe.
- Occasionally, a partial onset followed by a generalized seizure may identify the origin, for example, visual phenomena may suggest an occipital origin.
- Partial seizures may be associated with symptoms from their site of origin, for example, unilateral clonic movements from a frontal lesion, sensory symptoms from a parietal lesion.
- Postictal deficits from localized seizure activity may identify the site of origin of the seizures, for example, speech deficit from a dominant hemisphere onset seizure, postictal hemiparesis may indicate a frontal origin (also known as Todd's paralysis).

Differential Diagnosis in Diabetic Patients

- Hypoglycemia (generalized, occasionally focal)
- Nonketotic hyperosmolar coma (generalized or focal)
- Other metabolic abnormalities such as hyponatremia, hypomagnesemia, hypocalcemia, hepatic failure, and others (most often generalized)
- Cerebral venous thrombosis (generalized or focal)
- CNS infection including bacterial or fungal meningitis (generalized), cerebral abscess (focal with or without secondary generalization)
- Cerebral infarction or hemorrhage (usually suggests involvement of the cortex; focal onset)
- Cerebral tumor (focal onset)
- Congenital cerebral malformation, arteriovenous malformation (focal onset)
- Exacerbation of primary generalized epilepsy (often generalized)
- Recent or remote cerebral trauma (focal onset)
- Secondary to ethanol, street drugs (often generalized)
- Other

Investigation of Seizures

- Biochemistry: glucose, electrolytes, ammonia (if a history of hepatic disease), toxicology screen, calcium, magnesium.
- Unenhanced brain CT scan in the acute setting.
- Lumbar puncture (LP) if meningitis suspected; it may also be helpful in encephalitis and other conditions provided there is no contraindication such as raised intracranial pressure.
- EEG performed after postictal recovery or if it is suspected that there are ongoing seizures such as if "nonconvulsive status epilepticus" (ongoing seizures without tonic-clonic movements; NCSE).
- Sleep deprived EEG may be abnormal if standard EEG is normal.
- Brain MR is important in all new seizure patients to identify structural lesions not seen on the acute CT scan brain study (e.g., cortical dysplastic lesion, small tumors, vascular malformations) and to identify mesial temporal sclerosis.

Acute Treatment of Seizures

- Protect the airway by rolling the patient on his side, do not insert tongue blades or spoons into the mouth, loosen clothing around neck
- Protect the patient from self injury, remove from sources of injury
- Neck protection if patient has had a serious fall
- Check glucose level immediately

Status Epilepticus

- By convention SE is defined as greater than 30 minutes of continuous seizure activity or two or more sequential seizures without full recovery of consciousness; most generalized tonic-clonic seizures last 1 minute or less and complex partial seizures 2.5 minutes or less; seizures lasting more than 5 minutes without recovery of consciousness represent "impending SE" (24)

- ABCs—airway, breathing, circulation; may need to add oxygen; may need to intubate if ABCs unstable
- Check glucose level immediately
- Lorazepam intravenously (0.1 mg/kg) at 2 mg/min up to 8 mg preferred as initial therapy but is not definitive therapy because of the risk of recurrence (diazepam, an older choice, has a less predictable time course but can still be used rectally or intravenously; rectal dose is 10 to 20 mg in adults; IV dose is 10 to 20 mg; avoid repeated doses of diazepam)
- Phenytoin (or fosphenytoin if available, same dose) loaded as 20 mg/kg but infused no faster than 50 mg/min for regular phenytoin (150 mg/minute for fosphenytoin); Infuse *without* dextrose in the line; preferable to include ECG and blood pressure monitoring during the infusion; heart block is a contraindication to its use; in patients with SE taking phenytoin therapy as an outpatient, assume the blood level of phenytoin is negligible and administer a full loading dose; patients may exhibit nystagmus with therapeutic or higher levels of phenytoin
- Add thiamine 100 mg intravenously
- If SE continues despite the above, phenobarbital is the next choice (20 mg/kg intravenous loading dose at 50 mg/min). In some patients however, smaller intermittent doses added to phenytoin and lorazepam (e.g., 30–90 mg) may be sufficient to stop seizures; the combination of benzodiazepines and phenobarbital may precipitate respiratory depression—ICU consultation and readiness for intubation may be required; an alternative is IV valproic acid if available (40–60 mg/kg loading dose; 3 mg/kg/min) or IV levetiracetam (40 mg/kg)
- If SE continues despite the above, ICU admission highly likely: midazolam intravenous drip (0.2 mg/kg load then 0.75–10 µg/kg/min infusion) or propofol (with intubation, ventilation) [2 mg/kg load followed by 30–250 micrograms/kg/min]
- If SE continues additional options are high dose barbiturates or isoflurane anesthesia under continuous EEG control
- For suspected nonconvulsive SE (SE without tonic-clonic movements; presents with fluctuating confusion, fluctuating focal neurological deficits, may be a history of epilepsy or a known temporal lobe or frontal lesion) an urgent EEG is required;
- In typical tonic-clonic SE, an acute EEG is not always necessary (the beginning and end of seizures can be recognized clinically) but is helpful in some instances and in follow-up
- "Epilepsia partialis continua" refers to continuous focal seizures, for example, frontal lobe with continuous unilateral limb jerking

- Imaging workup includes an unenhanced CT head acutely; add CT venography (with cautions about contrast load) if cerebral venous thrombosis suspected, MR usually later; LP to exclude meningits

Chronic Management of Epilepsy

- Management similar in diabetics and nondiabetics.
- Avoidance of precipitating factors, sleep deprivation, ethanol and other forms of substance abuse.
- A single seizure in a patient with a normal neurological examination and normal investigations may not necessarily require antiepileptic medication.
- Requires ongoing neurological follow-up and a mechanism to follow antiepileptic drug levels, particularly if phenytoin is being used.
- When starting new therapy, slow upward titration of dosing is associated with fewer side effects.
- Adjust doses in renal failure if the drug is largely excreted by the kidney (e.g., gabapentin, pregabalin); use lower doses in elderly patients (non-metabolized and nonenzyme-inducing options may be preferable).
- Chronic therapy should be titrated to the individual and to their seizure diagnosis.
- Phenytoin, carbamazepine, phenobarbital (less frequently used) and primidone (contains phenobarbital) alter cytochrome p450 enzyme metabolism (enzyme inducers)—be cautious of potential interactions with diabetes medications; there is a possible relationship between valproic acid and increased insulin resistance.
- Gabapentin, levetiracetam, topiramate, zonisamide, lacosamide, pregabalin, and lamotrigine are not metabolized by p450.
- There are a large number of potential adverse effects, some dose and drug level related, from antiepileptic medications including neurological adverse effects; careful consultation with detailed pharmaceutical guidelines is recommended.
- Weight gain can occur from valproic acid, vigabatrin, gabapentin, and pregabalin, whereas topiramate and zonisamide are associated with weight loss.
- Special considerations exist for women of child bearing age, pregnant women, and lactating women with epilepsy; folate supplementation is mandatory during pregnancy, some agents may lower effectiveness of oral contraceptives; there are higher risks of fetal malformations with valproic acid.
- Reference (25)

Therapeutic Regimens for Seizures

- First line therapy for partial seizures: carbamazepine, lamotrigine, gabapentin, levetiracetam (not all guidelines include this agent), oxcarbazepine, topiramate, phenytoin (older agent).

- First line therapy for idiopathic generalized tonic-clonic seizures: lamotrigine, valproate, topiramate, levetiracetam.
- Absence epilepsy: ethosuximide, valproic acid.
- Refractory seizure add on medications: lacosamide, pregabalin, zonisamide, levetiracetam, clobazam.
- Phenytoin, carbamazepine, oxcarbazepine, or gabapentin can worsen myoclonus or absence seizures.
- Note that guidelines may differ among authors and change over time.
- References (26–29).

THE UNRESPONSIVE DIABETIC PATIENT

KEY POINTS

- Assume, treat, and check for hypoglycemia
- Patient may be postictal
- Immediate attention to ABCs
- Urgent imaging usually required when the patient is stabilized

Is the Patient Unresponsive?

- No response to voice, command; no eye opening to nail bed pressure or supraorbital pressure; patient does not actively resist eye opening

Immediate Management and Evaluation

- ABCs—airway, breathing, circulation, *glucose* level
- Establish an IV, give thiamine and 50% glucose unless a reliable glucose level is immediately available and is normal or elevated
- Neurological exam in a comatose patient

  Evidence of a head injury—bruises, Raccoon sign (blood around eye) suggests orbital fracture; Battle's sign is ecchymosis behind the ear from a basal skull fracture; hemotympanum, also secondary to a basal skull fracture
  Responsiveness (see Glasgow Coma Scale, Table 3.2)
  Pupils, dolls eyes (unless there is neck trauma requiring neck immobilization)
  Fundi, mouth and tympanic membrane
  Motor tone, spontaneous activity and withdrawal to nail bed pressure,
  Plantar responses and deep tendon reflexes
- Urgent unenhanced CT head scan
- Febrile and stiff neck, no focal signs—include lumbar puncture for meningitis

Differential Diagnosis

- Pupils reactive, no focal signs: metabolic-hypoglycemia, hypercalcemia, hyponatremia, postictal, hyperosmolar coma, toxins, drug intoxication,

Table 3.2 The Glasgow Coma Scale

Eye opening	
Spontaneous	4
To voice	3
To painful stimulation	2
None	1
Best verbal response	
Oriented	5
Confused	4
Inappropriate words	3
Unintelligible sounds	2
None	1
Best motor response	
Follows commands	6
Localizes pain	5
Withdraws from pain	4
Flexor response	3
Extensor response	2
None	1
Total	15

Note: 15 = normal.
Source: From Teasdale G, Jennett B. Assessment of coma and impaired consciousness. A practical scale. Lancet 1974; 2:81–84.

diffuse hypoxic-ischemic, meningitis, encephalitis, infection/sepsis; roving smooth conjugate eye movements help to suggest a diagnosis of metabolic encephalopathy.
- Pupils reactive, focal signs: cerebral (severe unilateral, or bilateral) or cerebellar infarction or hemorrhage, pontine or medullary infarct or hemorrhage, meningitis, encephalitis, hyperosmolar coma, hypoglycemia, infection/sepsis in a patient with preexisting neurological disease (MS, bilateral cerebral infarcts)
- Unreactive pupils: herniation secondary to cerebral or cerebellar infarction, hemorrhage or tumor, midbrain infarction, preexisting unreactive pupils (autonomic neuropathy or use of eye drops), severe barbiturate coma

VISUAL LOSS IN A DIABETIC

- Important to keep a wide differential diagnosis in patients with diabetes and new visual failure.
- New monocular visual loss requires urgent ophthalmological assessment; possibilities include deteriorated retinopathy, macular edema, vitreous

hemorrhage or detachment, retinal artery occlusion, endophthalmitis, anterior ischemic optic neuropathy (arteritic and nonarteritic), and others.

- Transient monocular visual loss may be secondary to amaurosis fugax; the visual loss is described as a sensation of a blind coming down over the visual field; ischemia to the retina from arteroembolism, most often from ipsilateral internal carotid artery stenosis and plaque.
- Optic neuritis presents with subacute monocular (rarely bilateral) central visual loss, with recovery over two to three weeks; may be a symptom of MS.
- Hemifield visual loss (or quadratic loss) involving both eyes indicates CNS damage to the visual system; patients unaware of this deficit may be involved in motor vehicle accidents.
- Bilateral visual blurring may occur during declines in control of glucose levels.
- "Transient obscuration of vision" or visual loss with bending, coughing, or straining may occur with raised intracranial pressure.

DIABETES AND DIZZINESS

- Exclude hypoglycemia, postural hypotension, canal cerumen (wax).
- Exclude hypotension secondary to new cardiac disease, cardiac arrhythmia.
- Evaluate relationship to initiation or escalation of pain pharmacotherapy (e.g., gabapentin, pregabalin, carbamazepine).
- True vertigo includes a sensation of movement or turning of self or the environment and most often is secondary to vestibular disease.
- Vertigo may be peripheral (vestibular) or central (CNS cause); isolated vertigo is an uncommon symptom of cerebral ischemia.
- Patients may refer to unsteadiness (from sensory loss, motor weakness, cerebral infarction) as dizziness—clarify during the history taking.

DIPLOPLIA IN A DIABETIC PATIENT

- Diploplia from weakness of an eye muscle disappears when one eye is covered.
- Ischemic third nerve palsy, weakness of levator palpebrae, medial rectus, superior and inferior rectus: unilateral ptosis, impaired upgaze, downgaze and medial gaze; pupillary sparing is usually found in diabetics with this condition.
- Ischemic sixth nerve palsy presents with weakness of the lateral rectus muscle: lateral separation of images, worse in looking toward the side of the palsy, worse looking in the distance; when covering up the eye that has the weak lateral rectus muscle, the image that disappears should be more eccentric (more lateral).

- Sixth nerve palsies are associated with raised intracranial pressure and have been called "false localizing signs."
- Monocular diploplia (does not go away from covering one eye) from temporal lobe cerebral disease is uncommon.
- Lacunar infarction of the brain stem may present with diploplia from damage to the third cranial nerve nucleus (midbrain) or sixth cranial nerve nucleus (pons) or their axons as they exit the brain stem.
- The medial longitudinal fasciculus, connecting the third and sixth cranial nuclei may be damaged by a lacunar infarction causing internuclear ophthalmoplegia (INO); INO is manifest as weakness of adduction of the eye on the side of the brain stem lesion and lateral nystagmus of the opposite, or abducting eye; some forms involve the pupillary reaction and are called "'anterior" INO from a midbrain lesion.
- The "one and a half" syndrome, from a pontine infarction, has complete loss of horizontal movement in one eye and preserved abduction in the other eye.
- Myasthenia gravis presents with fatiguable eye muscle weakness (fluctuates, worse later in the day) and includes bilateral signs, ptosis; pupils are not involved; early disease may have ptosis only.
- Imaging studies are required to exclude structural lesions. MR imaging is preferred when a brain stem or posterior fossa lesion is suspected.

SPEECH DISTURBANCE IN A DIABETIC PATIENT

- Dysarthria refers to an abnormality of speech articulation; patients with dysarthria have slurring of speech but intact language with intact understanding and the appropriate use of words; dysarthria may involve mouth, tongue, or palate movement (see chap. 2).
- Dysarthria may occur from a diffuse metabolic disturbance including hypoglycemia and hyperglycemia; right hemisphere or pontine infarction or other types of damage; use of sedative or opioid medications, ethanol or street drugs; weakness of facial, tongue, or palate muscles from ALS, myasthenia gravis, other neuromuscular conditions.
- Aphasia (also called dysphasia) is a disorder of the dominant cortex, usually the left hemisphere that involves language function.
- Aphasia may involve the production of speech (motor or Broca's aphasia involving the posterior inferior frontal lobe near the medial insula) or the reception of speech (sensory aphasia or Wernicke's aphasia involving the posterior temporal lobe) or both (global aphasia); writing is also involved.
- Motor aphasia is characterized by inability to make normal words and sentences, often associated with acute frustration; patients may speak short phrases repetitively in an attempt to speak; in milder motor aphasia, words or letters may be used inappropriately (paraphasic errors); motor aphasia is often termed "nonfluent."

- Sensory aphasia is characterized by lack of comprehension, inability to repeat and fluent nonsensical speech with errors of words and letters (paraphasic errors).
- Other rare aphasias are described: conduction aphasia impairs the ability to repeat speech but comprehension and speech output are intact; transcortical motor aphasia or sensory aphasia have preserved repetition but impaired motor and sensory speech function respectively; nominal aphasia impairs naming.
- Aphasia in a diabetic patient may be secondary to a stroke, may be postictal following a focal seizure, or arise from other intracranial causes; patients with hypoglycemia and nonketotic hyperosmolar syndrome may have aphasia.
- Mutism may arise from severe dysarthria, global aphasia, bilateral frontal lobe disease, or a conversion psychiatric disorder.

ATAXIA OF GAIT IN A DIABETIC PATIENT

- Ataxia refers to an inability to coordinate normal muscle movements
- Gait unsteadiness may have a number of causes: spinal, hip, or leg pain, muscle paralysis from motor neuropathy, spinal cord, cerebellar or frontal lobe disease, loss of proprioceptive sensation in the legs, neuropathic pain in the feet, foot drop, lumbosacral plexopathy
- A complete neurological examination is required to localize the cause of ataxia
- Inability to maintain stance with eye closure suggests an abnormality of proprioception, secondary to loss or demyelination of sensory axons in polyneuropathy, or loss or demyelination of axons in the dorsal columns of the spinal cord
- In diabetic patients, common causes of gait ataxia are sensory polyneuropathy (loss of proprioception, loss of pressure sensation on the sole), bifrontal cerebral infarcts, or midline cerebellar lacunar infarcts.
- Multiple bilateral lacunar infarcts ("etat lacunaire") are associated with gait ataxia, dementia, dysarthria, dysphagia (difficulty swallowing), and urinary incontinence

HEADACHES AND DIABETES

- Headache is a common neurological symptom; a careful history is often sufficient to distinguish the type of headache.
- New or different headaches are especially important to evaluate.
- A new headache may be a symptom of either hyperglycemia or hypoglycemia.
- Common headaches, unrelated to diabetes, include migraine and tension-type headaches (see Table 3.3 for diagnostic criteria from the International Headache Society).

Table 3.3 Abbreviated Key Points of the International Headache Classification-2

Primary headaches
Migraine
Migraine without aura diagnostic criteria:
A. At least 5 attacks fulfilling criteria B–D
B. Headache attacks lasting 4–72 hr (untreated or unsuccessfully treated)
C. Headache has at least two of the following characteristics:
    1. Unilateral location
    2. Pulsating quality
    3. Moderate or severe pain intensity
    4. Aggravation by or causing avoidance of routine physical activity (e.g., walking or climbing stairs)
D. During headache at least one of the following:
    1. Nausea and/or vomiting
    2. Photophobia and phonophobia
E. Not attributed to another disorder

Headache with aura diagnostic criteria:
A. At least two attacks fulfilling criterion B
B. Migraine aura fulfilling criteria B and C for one of the subforms
C. Not attributed to another disorder

Typical aura diagnostic criteria:
A. At least 2 attacks fulfilling criteria B–D
B. Aura consisting of at least one of the following, but no motor weakness:
    1. Fully reversible visual symptoms including positive features (e.g., flickering lights, spots, or lines) and/or negative features (i.e., loss of vision)
    2. Fully reversible sensory symptoms including positive features (i.e., pins and needles) and/or negative features (i.e., numbness)
    3. Fully reversible dysphasic speech disturbance
C. At least two of the following:
    1. Homonymous visual symptoms and/or unilateral sensory symptoms
    2. At least one aura symptom develops gradually over ≥ 5 minutes and/or different aura symptoms occur in succession over ≥ 5 minutes
    3. Each symptom lasts ≥ 5 and ≤ 60 minutes
D. Headache fulfilling criteria for migraine without aura begins during the aura or follows aura within 60 minutes
E. Not attributed to another disorder

Tension-type headache
Frequent episodic tension-type headache diagnostic criteria:
A. At least 10 episodes occurring on ≥ 1 but < 15 days/mo for at least 3 mo (≥ 12 and < 180 days/yr) and fulfilling criteria B–D
B. Headache lasting from 30 minutes to 7 days
C. Headache has at least two of the following characteristics:
    1. bilateral location
    2. pressing/tightening (non-pulsating) quality
    3. mild or moderate intensity
    4. not aggravated by routine physical activity such as walking or climbing stairs

(Continued)

Table 3.3 Abbreviated Key Points of the International Headache Classification-2 (*Continued*)

D. Both of the following:
    1. no nausea or vomiting (anorexia may occur)
    2. no more than one of photophobia or phonophobia
E. Not attributed to another disorder

Chronic tension-type headache diagnostic criteria:
A. Headache occurring on ≥15 days/mo on average for >3 mo (≥180 days/yr) and fulfilling criteria B–D
B. Headache lasts hours or may be continuous
C. Headache has at least two of the following characteristics:
    1. Bilateral location
    2. Pressing/tightening (nonpulsating) quality
    3. Mild or moderate intensity
    4. Not aggravated by routine physical activity such as walking or climbing stairs
D. Both of the following:
    1. No more than one of photophobia, phonophobia, or mild nausea
    2. No moderate or severe nausea or vomiting
E. Not attributed to another disorder

Cluster headache and other trigeminal autonomic cephalgias
Other primary headaches
Secondary headaches
Headache attributed to head and/or neck trauma
Headache attributed to cranial or cervical vascular disorder
Headache attributed to nonvascular intracranial disorder
Headache attributed to a substance or its withdrawal
Headache attributed to infection
Headache attributed to disorders of homeostasis
Headache or facial pain attributed to disorder of cranium, neck, eyes, ears, nose, sinuses, teeth, mouth, or other facial or cranial structures
Headache attributed to psychiatric disorder
Cranial neuralgias, facial pain, and other headaches

Source: Reproduced and summarized with permission of International Headache Society. Please refer to The International Classification of Headache Disorders, 2nd ed. Cephalalgia 2004; 24(suppl 1) for full details. Available at: http://ihs-classification.org/en/.

- Migraine headaches often develop in childhood, adolescence, or young adulthood and are associated with a family history of headache; they are often unilateral, pounding, sometimes very severe and are associated with photphobia and phonophobia, nausea or vomiting; they last 4 to 72 hours; many migraine headaches are associated with an aura: bright flashing lights, flickering lights, "lightning bolts" ("scintillating scotomata"), slowly spreading unilateral tingling sensations or, less commonly, loss of vision, loss of sensation, motor weakness, speech disturbance, or altered level of consciousness (LOC).

- Hypoglycemia can trigger migraine headaches.
- Migraine therapy includes prophylactic agents to prevent frequent headaches (e.g., β-blockers, amitryptilene, topiramate, others) or abortive agents to reverse a severe attack (e.g., triptan or ergotamine medications).
- Risks of migraine therapy in diabetic patients: β-Blockers may mask symptoms of hypoglycemia; amitryptilene may exacerbate abnormalities of bladder emptying; triptans and ergots are contraindicated in patients with cardiovascular disease.
- Tension-type headaches, previously called muscle contraction headaches, may develop at any age, and are often bilateral, persistent with dull frontotemporal or occipitocervical pain and not associated with nausea, vomiting or aura.
- Secondary headaches are headaches from other causes such as intracranial tumors, skull lesions, cervical spondylosis, and many others.
- Headaches are common in cerebral infarction and hemorrhage (stroke).
- Cerebral venous thrombosis is more common in diabetics than nondiabetics and may present with severe headache, nausea, and vomiting with or without focal neurological signs and symptoms.
- Headaches are common following a generalized seizure.
- "Red flag" headaches: (*i*) Raised intracranial pressure (ICP): mild or moderate bilateral headache, worse in morning, worse with bending over or coughing, with or without transient visual loss ("transient obscuration of vision"), with or without sixth cranial nerve weakness, papilledema or focal neurological signs; raised ICP is secondary to mass lesions (tumors, abscesses, hemorrhage, others), hydrocephalus, trauma or benign intracranial hypertension; (*ii*) "thunderclap" headache: sudden onset during sleep, sexual intercourse or exercise and described by the patient as a new headache, "the worst headache of my life"; this headache may be associated with subarachnoid hemorrhage from a ruptured berry aneurysm or arteriovenous malformation, from cerebral infarction, from vertebral or carotid artery dissection, or from cerebral venous thrombosis; patients with subarachnoid hemorrhage may have a stiff neck (meningismus) and subvitreous hemorrhages on funduscopic examination; (*iii*) temporal arteritis headache: unilateral temporal headache in an older person, may be associated with temporal artery tenderness, weight loss, malaise, and an elevated erythrocyte sedimentation rate; (*iv*) headache with meningitis: subacute bilateral headache with neck stiffness, fever, malaise, decreased LOC, sometimes focal signs; neck pain from extending the knee when the patient is supine with their hip and knee flexed (Kernig's sign) or knee and hip flexion on bending the head (Brudzinski's sign).

DEMENTIA IN A DIABETIC PATIENT

KEY POINTS

- Dementia refers to cognitive dysfunction in two or more areas of brain function, such as memory and executive function, that interferes with social functioning at home or work.
- The diagnosis requires input from a witness: spouse, other relative, friend.
- Dementia can be mimicked by severe depression or use of medications.
- "Beclouded" dementia refers to acute confusion in a patient hospitalized for a separate systemic illness.
- Essential to check for signs of other neurological disorders.

History

Are There Symptoms of Memory Loss or Other Cognitive Difficulties?

- Ask about problems with remembering names or events, repeating stories or questions, lost or wandering behavior, and kitchen accidents (e.g., stove left on).
- A corroborative history from a witness is critical—when insight is impaired, the severity of the symptoms may be dramatically underestimated by the patient. Conversely, if the witness is unaware of these symptoms then benign forgetfulness, rather than dementia, may be present.

Are the Cognitive Symptoms Associated with Functional Limitations?

- Ask about finances, shopping, use of telephone, cooking, housework, driving. Is there anything the patient used to do but now cannot do because of the cognitive symptoms? Could the patient take care of him/herself if left alone for a week?

What is the Time Course of the Symptoms?

- Sudden onset, a course of stepwise deteriorations, or sudden onset without further progression can be seen in vascular dementia. A relatively smooth progressive course is seen in most neurodegenerative diseases. Wide fluctuations in level of consciousness can be seen in Lewy body dementia. A rapidly progressive course over weeks or months raises the possibility of a prion disease, vasculitis or paraneoplastic syndrome. Impairment with fluctuating alertness that is reversible suggests a delirium rather than a dementia.

Is There a History of Stroke? Are There Vascular Risk Factors?

- Suggests the possibility of vascular dementia. Vascular risk factors have been associated with both vascular dementia and Alzheimer's disease.

Are There Motor or Gait Symptoms?

- Slowed gait, falls, hypophonia or bradykinesia raise the possibility of a Parkinson's plus syndrome, cerebrovascular disease, normal pressure hydrocephalus or associated motor neuron disease.

Is There a Sleep Disturbance?

- REM sleep behavior disorder, marked by preserved limb movements during the REM sleep phase, can precede or accompany the onset of Parkinson's disease or Alzheimer's disease. The patient may be unaware of the symptoms, but it can be elicited by history from a witness or bed partner.

What Medications is the Patient Taking?

- The elderly are vulnerable to cognitive side effects of psychoactive medications such as benzodiazepines.

Are There Symptoms of Depression or Another Psychiatric Disorder?

- Rarely, severe depression in the elderly can present as a "pseudodementia." More commonly, depression or adjustment disorder can occur in the early stages of dementia when insight is preserved. Identification and treatment of coexisting depression may improve quality of life.

Neurological Examination

- Mental status examination should be performed to interrogate the following mental functions (at minimum): orientation, delayed recall, attention and working memory, calculation, visuospatial construction, and language
  - Brief (5–10 minute) global cognitive screening tests have been developed to assess these functions; perhaps the most widely used are the Montreal Cognitive Assessment Tool (MoCA; Table 2.2) and the Mini-Mental Status Examination (MMSE). We recommend the MoCA.
- The pattern of dysfunction across the cognitive domains can suggest the underlying neuropathology, particularly if the patient is examined relatively early in the course of the disease before deficits become more severe and widespread
  - Poor orientation and impaired delayed recall suggests Alzheimer's disease.
  - Psychomotor slowing, decreased attention, and reduced working memory suggests vascular dementia or normal pressure hydrocephalus.
  - Language impairment suggests a primary progressive aphasia.
  - Behavioral disturbances, inappropriate joking, or sexual behavior suggests frontotemporal dementia.
  - Visuospatial dysfunction suggests Lewy body dementia.

- Parkinsonian signs (rigidity, stooped shuffling gait): Parkinson's disease or a Parkinson's plus syndrome (Lewy body disease, progressive supranuclear palsy, corticobasal degeneration, multiple system atrophy).
- Vertical gaze palsy, axial rigidity: progressive supranuclear palsy.
- Severe unilateral apraxia or alien limb phenomenon: corticobasal degeneration.
- Magnetic gait, incontinence: normal pressure hydrocephalus.
- Orthostatic hypotension to other autonomic signs: multiple system atrophy.
- Focal neurological signs: symptomatic or asymptomatic stroke (cerebral infarction) that may be related to the cognitive symptoms.

Investigations

- Vitamin B_{12}, thyroid-stimulating hormone: B_{12} deficiency and hypothyroidism can cause dementia and are readily correctable.
- Testing for syphilis (VDRL, rapid plasmin reagin): not recommended by guidelines for all cases, but should be considered in higher-risk groups.
- Neuroimaging: recommended in new-onset dementia to rule out potentially treatable conditions such as frontal brain tumor (rare), silent stroke or white matter lesions ("leukoaraiosis"), and normal pressure hydrocephalus. Even when treatable causes are not found, neuroimaging may give prognostic information by suggesting the underlying neuropathologic cause based on patterns of brain volume loss: frontotemporal lobes—frontotemporal dementia, medial temporal lobes—Alzheimer's disease, midbrain—progressive supranuclear palsy. Either MRI or CT are adequate; however MRI gives better anatomic resolution and may be more sensitive for brain atrophy.
- Lumbar puncture: should be considered in cases of rapidly progressive dementia: routine tests (protein, glucose, cell count) as well as 14-3-3 protein (elevated in Creutzfeldt–Jakob disease and encephalitis), paraneoplastic antibodies, VDRL, and cytology as appropriate.
- Electroencephalography: not helpful in most cases. Consider when there is intermittent cognitive impairment (to rule out complex partial seizures), when NCSE is suspected or when a Creutzfeldt–Jakob disease is suspected (to look for the typical periodic sharp waves seen in the disease).
- Nuclear medicine: PET or SPECT can be used to look for regions of hypometabolism or decreased blood flow that correlate with brain regions involved by the neuropathology. Biparietal hypometabolism is usually seen in cases of AD and frontotemporal hypometabolism is seen in frontotemporal dementia.

4

"Red flags" in neurology and diabetes

In this chapter we identify a series of "red flags," issues of immediate clinical concern that are important for both neurologists and diabetologists. While listed as important points for consideration here, some of the topics have expanded discussion in further chapters in the book.

KEY POINTS

- A restless, confused type 1 diabetic patient may have diabetic ketoacidosis
- Focal signs, seizures, confusion in a type 2 diabetic patient may indicate hyperosmolar syndrome
- Pain from myocardial ischemia, pulmonary embolism or abdominal emergencies may be masked in diabetic patients
- Upper motor neuron signs may be masked in diabetic patients
- Assess all diabetic patients for foot ulcers
- Angiographic dye can precipitate acute renal failure in diabetic patients
- Screen new patients with TIAs or cerebral infarcts for undiagnosed type 2 diabetes mellitus

DIABETIC KETOACIDOSIS

- A medical/diabetic emergency (see also chap. 5)
- Typically a type 1 diabetic patient but type 2 may also present this way
- Precipitated by infection, interruption of insulin use, trauma, myocardial infarction, pregnancy or other causes
- May present with loss of appetite, intercurrent infection, thirst, polyuria, weight loss, dyspnea (labored respiration-Kussmaul respiration; fruity odor on breath), drowsiness and fatigue, vague abdominal pain, sometimes coma

- Laboratory diagnosis: anion gap metabolic acidosis, serum ketonemia (with ketonuria), usually elevated glucose, other electrolye abnormalities
- Urgent rehydration, treatment of electrolyte abnormalities, control of hyperglycemia is essential, insulin therapy when the patient is eukalemic

NONKETOTIC DIABETIC HYPEROSMOLAR SYNDROME

- A medical/diabetic emergency (see chap. 5) with a high mortality rate
- Usually in an older, type 2 diabetic patient and often precipitated by infection
- May present with altered level of consciousness, focal neurological signs, or seizures
- Urgent rehydration, treatment of electrolyte abnormalties, and control of hyperglycemia are essential
- Antiepileptic agents may not be required if seizures are isolated and only occur in the acute stage

CLOUDED NEUROLOGICAL SIGNS

Clouding of Pain

- "Silent" or painless myocardial infarction or angina; secondary to loss of cardiac sensory nerves (from diabetic neuropathy)
- Silent pulmonary embolism
- Silent acute abdomen without abdominal rigidity; from loss of visceral sensation secondary to neuropathy and loss of abdominal innervation from truncal motor neuropathy: silent appendicitis, bowel obstruction (increased risk in diabetes from constipation), diverticular disease, bowel ischemia (increased risk in patients with diabetes-related atherosclerosis), bowel perforation
- Urinary tract infections (increased risk with atonic bladders and indwelling catheters)

Loss of sensation in the heart or abdominal viscera from diabetic neuropathy may result in painless medical emergencies. To diagnose unexpected cardiac ischemia (may occur in patients following stroke) a routine EKG is indicated at the time of their neurological presentation. If there is a suspicion of myocardial infarction, troponin T or I levels are indicated. Unexpected signs or findings suggesting the possibility of a cardiac emergency include new hypotension, tachycardia, shortness of breath, arrhythmia, a sudden change in glucose control, elevated CK levels, and abnormal segmental cardiac wall movement on a screening (for embolic sources of stroke) 2-D echocardiogram. Patients admitted with cerebral ischemia (TIA or infarction) associated with apparent new onset atrial fibrillation should be screened for an underlying myocardial infarction.

Failure to recognize an abdominal emergency may occur in diabetic patients because of loss of visceral sensation and failure to generate acute abdominal muscle contractions (rigidity or guarding). This may be exacerbated in patients with additional neurological disease including spinal cord injury, cerebral infarction and other problems. Diabetic patients with acute on chronic constipation are at risk for unrecognized bowel perforation and peritonitis.

Absence of Upper Motor Neuron Signs

- Neurological signs of an upper motor neuron lesion may be obscured by diabetic neuropathy
- An absent plantar response may occur because of toe paralysis from peroneal neuropathy or polyneuropathy
- Masking of hyperreflexia (from polyneuropathy)
- Masking of spasticity from hypotonia secondary to muscle weakness

Loss of typical upper motor neuron signs of central nervous system disease may mislead examiners in their assessment of the cause and potential treatment of new neurological problems. Since an upper motor neuron sign requires an intact reflex loop (sensation of the stimulus from the reflex hammer, intact sensory organs and nerves, normal spinal cord synapses and normal motor output), subtle neuropathy that interrupts any component of the reflex loop may interrupt the sign. Patients with acute spinal cord problems may present with diffuse weakness, but they may have flaccid arreflexic paralysis erroneously suggesting GBS. In patients with concurrent polyneuropathy, stocking and glove sensory alterations may also cloud the exact localization of a separate neuro-logical problem. Vigilance in diabetic patients for potential spinal cord disease is important because upper motor neuron signs and a sensory level may be difficult to identify.

RISKS FROM CONTRAST AGENTS

- Risk of nephrotoxicity from iodinated contrast agents used for cerebral angiography, CT angiography; defined as a 25% rise in serum creatinine.
- Incidence in diabetes mellitus ranges from 6% to 30% (risk of renal failure requiring dialysis much lower); increased risk in patients with glucose intolerance; risk in diabetic patients with creatinine of greater than 354 μmol/L (4.0 mg%) may be as high as 80% but there is also an increased risk with normal renal function.
- In addition to diabetes, risk factors for contrast nephropathy are: age >75, heart failure, cirrhosis, hypovolemia, surgery, arterial catheterization, atherosclerosis and renal emboli, hypertension, hypotension, nonsteroidal anti-inflammatory agents, use of intra-aortic balloon pump, low serum albumin, renal transplantation, anemia, other nephrotoxins (e.g.,

aminoglycosides, cyclosporine, cisplatinum), preexisiting renal disease and proteinuria.
- Risk factors are synergistic when combined.
- Larger doses of contrast agents are more toxic (>5 mL × kg of body weight/creatinine in mg%); higher-osmolar iodine contrast is more toxic than a lower-osmolar agent.
- Rises in creatinine from nephropathy peak at 3 days and subside by 10 days following contrast administration.
- Check creatinine, or creatinine clearance before procedure.
- Prevent nephropathy by administering precontrast intravenous isotonic saline (1 mL/kg/hr for 12 hours before procedure and 12 hours post procedure); there is a possible benefit from N-acetylcysteine in preventing contrast nephropathy but the data are not conclusive.
- Withold other nephrotoxins if possible. Metformin should be held 48 hours pre procedure when there is a concern about acidosis in the setting of contrast induced nephropathy and renal dysfunction and resumed if there is no rise in creatinine; beware of diabetes decompensation from holding metformin.
- Low or iso-osmolar agents may be the safest agents to use in diabetic patients, but the evidence for their benefit is incomplete; other agents for the treatment or prevention of contrast nephropathy are of uncertain benefit; Forced diuresis or bicarbonate diuresis are not recommended.
- References (30,31).

UNRECOGNIZED POOR OUTPATIENT CONTROL
- May be difficult to judge during an inpatient hospitalization
- Review outpatient glycemia diaries in patients admitted to hospital
- Discuss ongoing management with the patient's outpatient diabetes caregivers; refer if necessary
- HbA1c may predict level of chronic glucose control

CHRONIC DIABETES MANAGEMENT
- Multidisciplinary care is essential to optimal long-term diabetes care
- Follow-up requires an identified regular care manager, setting defined goals, appropriate cost-effective testing, and careful attention toward hypoglycemia

The Primacy of Multidisciplinary Teams
- As a chronic disease that typically becomes more complex and clinically problematic over time, comprehensive management usually taxes the skill and time set of a single practitioner.

- A nurse manager or diabetes educator should be involved for regular visits to enhance disease understanding, adherence to therapy and assist with scheduling routine screening tests.
- A dietician with experience in diabetes is frequently needed, especially if the patient is on multi injection insulin using specific carbohydrate counts for dosing.
- A social worker/psychologist team is frequently required; depression and other psychological stressors are common among persons with diabetes and in some cases (e.g., post myocardial infarction) may be strong predictors of mortality. The success of chronic disease management depends on attention toward coexisting social/psychological/psychiatric comorbidities.

Five Major Barriers to Successful Diabetes Medical Follow-Up

Lack of an Identified Primary Diabetes Manager and/or Infrequent Clinical Follow-Up Visits

- Many persons with diabetes periodically require more frequent monthly or bimonthly follow-up clinical visits. This should be made available through the diabetes team with the understanding that the primary diabetes physician will oversee the team actions.
- "Lost to follow-up" is a common antecedent to a major diabetes complication or decompensation event.

Lack of a Defined and Achievable Goal

- Many patients are subject to a massive "information download" during their prescribed diabetes education visits. There is often perceived pressure to "fix everything" all at once commonly leading to frustration and failure.
- An achievable individualized goal should be defined in a given time-frame and assessed at subsequent follow-up visits. This may be as simple as learning to test a capillary glucose once a day or as complex as determining the necessary basal rate overnight on an insulin pump.

Overemphasis on Capillary Glucose Testing in Type 2 Diabetes

- For persons with type 2 diabetes not on insulin, the bulk of the literature shows that self-glucose monitoring does not improve overall glycemic control or quality of life (32,33). At roughly $1.00 per glucometer strip, this represents a potentially enormous expenditure for little benefit.
- A preferred approach may be glucose monitoring for a limited time interval such as two weeks prior to a team visit or prior to a major change in therapy.

Capillary Glucose Results Are Not Reviewed

- Many persons with diabetes do extensive glucose monitoring because they are so instructed but their results may not be carefully or extensively assessed by the patient or physician. Although capillary glucose testing can be useful for immediate management decisions, the patient must understand the impact of insulin kinetics, diet content, activity levels and illness to make correct decisions.
- Long-term monitoring data is a valuable source of information that may disclose patterns of insulin administration errors, hypoglycemic precipitants and other issues. This exercise involves considerable work and ideally, is best accomplished by the patient analyzing their own glucose records every two to four weeks.
- The diabetes team's role is to shift the responsibility for self-assessment to the able patient who must be willing and equipped to assume this aspect of their care.

Lack of Attention to Hypoglycemia

- Hypoglycemia, particularly severe hypoglycemia, increases in frequency as diabetes control improves, especially toward a HbA1c target range of 6.5% to 7.0% (34).
- Hypoglycemia is a particularly unpleasant experience that can result in situations ranging from social embarrassment to death.
- Fear of hypoglycemia is a common reason for patient reluctance to revise their diabetes management plan and for failure to improve hyperglycemia; Full disclosure by patients to the team and attention to these concerns by the team are critical to a collaborative therapeutic relationship.
- Optimum individual diabetes control depends on what is achievable with a minimum of hypoglycemia (see chap. 1).

Conclusions

- Complex chronic diabetes medical management should include attention by specialists to specific complications while a designated physician or team be responsible for remaining issues and overall management.
- References (32,33).

PAIN PHARMACOTHERAPY AND DIABETIC NEPHROPATHY

- Avoid nonsteroidal anti-inflammatory medications (NSAIDs) in patients with diabetic nephropathy; their efficacy in neuropathic pain is not established.

- Gabapentin and pregabalin are renally excreted but can be used in patients with renal failure at a lower dose (refer to pharmaceutical guidelines).
- Urinary retention can develop from agents with anticholinergic properties (e.g., amitryptilene and relatives).
- There are rare reports of renal failure secondary to carbamazepine, lamotrigine.
- Topiramate has reduced clearance in severe renal failure; associated with renal calculi.

FOOT ULCERATION

- Foot ulceration is a medical emergency because of the risks of deep infection and osteomyelitis.
- Patients with foot ulcers are at significant risk for amputation.
- May be provoked by minor trauma, poorly fitting footware, or lack of injury awareness.
- Patients with polyneuropathy at increased risk for foot ulceration, and may be unaware of its presence.
- Insensitivity to injury and poor healing from sensory polyneuropathy and foot deformity from muscle denervation (neuropathy involving motor axons) predispose to ulceration.
- Other risk factors are macrovascular and microvascular disease, and predisposition to infection.
- Urgent referral to diabetic foot care clinic is indicated; stopping weight bearing, removal of offending footware or braces, sometimes a "walking cast" is required, aggressive treatment of infection, overall multidisciplinary management.
- Prevention involves regular clinic foot examination, daily individual foot inspection, regular professional callus debridement, and smoking cessation.

GLUCOCORTICOIDS (CORTICOSTEROIDS) IN DIABETIC PATIENTS

- Glucocorticoid therapy can be associated with the development of ketoacidosis or hyperosmolar coma in patients already known to have diabetes or in patients without a previous diagnosis.
- The incidence of "steroid diabetes" ranges from 1% to 46% of those treated with glucocorticoids; 40% in patients with renal disease.
- Initiation of glucocorticoids in diabetes requires a strategy to detect, monitor and aggressively treat hyperglycemia.
- Patients rendered euglycemic with intensified therapy for diabetes during glucocorticoid treatment may develop hypoglycemia when glucocorticoids are tapered or stopped.

- Patients at risk for the development of overt diabetes mellitus from glucocorticoid use include those with impaired fasting glucose, impaired glucose tolerance or a history of gestational diabetes; advanced age and hypercholesterolemia are additional risk factors.
- Monitor blood glucose every one to two weeks in patients at risk for steroid diabetes; test second void preprandial urine twice daily initially then thrice weekly; if glycosuria is detected, blood sampling is required to confirm the diagnosis.
- Short-term glucocorticoid regimens (<2 weeks) may simply require monitoring only; longer-term glucocorticoid regimens may require more aggressive therapy (e.g., addition of insulin or increase in insulin dosing).
- Oral therapy usually insufficient for uncontrolled steroid diabetes.
- References (35–37).

USE OF INTRAVENOUS γ GLOBULIN IN DIABETIC PATIENTS

- Caution is required in diabetic patients; intravenous γ globulin (IVIG) protein load may theoretically exacerbate diabetic nephropathy.
- Slower infusion rates may be indicated.
- There is an increased risk of thrombogenesis: myocardial infarction, TIA or cerebral infarction, deep venous thrombosis, pulmonary emboli, and renal artery thrombosis.
- Other risk factors for thromboembolic events using IVIG are: advanced age, known atherosclerosis, previous thromboembolic events, excessive dose, or overly rapid infusion.
- Do not withhold IVIG (including chronic therapy) from diabetics with firm indications: GBS, CIDP, MG, and others.
- Diabetes is a risk factor for rare acute renal failure secondary to IVIG: other risk factors are older age, additional nephrotoxin useage, hypovolemia, preexisting renal failure (35).

RECOGNIZING NEUROPATHIC PAIN

- Described as burning, tingling, prickling, "pins and needles," tight sensations, and episodic electrical jolts.
- May be "stocking and glove" in distribution in polyneuropathy or in a specific nerve territory in focal neuropathies (e.g., thumb, index, middle finger and palm in carpal tunnel syndrome).
- May be worse at night; patients with carpal tunnel syndrome have more prominent symptoms at night or on awakening.
- May be provoked by innocuous stimuli (allodynia) such as bed covers.
- Check that footware is loose and not causing injury; inspect feet.

- Consider pharmacotherapy and start with a low dose such as before bedtime: gabapentin, pregabalin, amitryptiline, nortriptilene, duloxetine, tramacet, others.
- Truncal neuropathy may be mistaken for a thoracic or abdominal emergency but is distinguished by neuropathic pain descriptors; the pain radiates from the back around chest or abdomen in several contiguous dermatomes resembling herpes zoster without a rash; there is often an area of sensory loss (see chap. 10).
- Severe thigh and proximal leg pain may indicate the development of lumbosacral plexopathy.

Neuropathic pain is important to ask about, evaluate and treat whenever diabetic patients are encountered. A history of pain symptoms, their distribution and their tolerance of previous analgesia is required as part of the evaluation. If the pain is stocking or lower limb in distribution, inspect the feet and at minimum perform a screening lower limb neurological examination (see chap. 2).

RECOGNIZING TIAS

- Cardinal symptoms of TIA are as follows:
  - Acute weakness with loss of power on one side (face, arm, and leg)
  - Acute aphasia with loss of speech or ability to understand speech or writing
  - Acute loss of vision in one hemi-field or one eye
- May be ignored by patients or clinicians because of preexisting neuropathy, carpal tunnel syndrome, abnormal gait.
- Other symptoms such as acute clumsiness, sensory loss beyond a single nerve territory, change in gait, or diploplia could all represent possible cerebral infarction or TIA. Key features are a sudden onset and maximal deficit at onset.
- TIAs by definition clear within 24 hours but most last less than an hour; there should be no residual symptoms, persistent deficit on examination or an imaging abnormality all of which suggest cerebral infarction (identified by brain CT or MR).
- Transient neurological symptoms may indicate a cerebral infarction rather than a TIA when there is imaging evidence of damage. This can be predicted by the presence of residual symptoms despite a normal examination.
- TIAs require urgent investigation, especially if there is motor involvement, change in speech: possible hospitalization, acute imaging (CT with or without CT angiography), evaluation of cartotid arteries by CTA or ultrasound, ECG to identify atrial fibrillation, blood hematology to identify thrombocytosis, 2-D echocardiography to exclude a cardiac source of cerebral embolism.

RECOGNIZING SEIZURES

- A nocturnal seizure may indicate unrecognized hypoglycemia.
- Bed partner may be helpful in identifying whether a seizure has taken place.
- On awakening patient may note mouth or tongue damage from biting, painful muscles, urinary or bowel incontinence and rarely lumbar or other fractures from self injury.
- Some forms of epilepsy are exclusively nocturnal. A full neurological workup is indicated.
- Driving privileges may be retained, after a period of observation, if a seizure is recognized to be secondary to hypoglycemia and appropriate adjustments in glycemic control are made.

THIAMINE AND GLUCOSE INFUSIONS

- Include thiamine (100 mg IV) to accompany all acute glucose infusions.
- Do not attempt to replace thiamine orally since absorption is inadequate by this route.
- There is a risk of Wernicke-Korsakoff disease from glucose infusions without thiamine.

HYPOGLYCEMIC UNAWARENESS

- Hypoglycemia is defined as a plasma glucose concentration below 2.7 mmol/L (50 mg/dL).
- Symptoms of hypoglycemia from rises in counter-regulatory hormones may begin at glucose levels of 4.0 mmol/L (70 mg/dL).
- Cognitive function begins to decline below 2.7 mmol/L, although patients with a history of hypoglycemia may be resistant. Patients with chronic hyperglycemia may experience symptoms of hypoglycemia at higher glucose levels.
- As a result of cognitive dysfunction, and glucagon levels (to counteract declines in glucose) that fail to rise, patients may become seriously impaired without realizing it and fail to take adequate protective measures.
- Recurrent hypoglycemia may also contribute to an increased risk of hypoglycemic unawareness; control of hypoglycemia restores the sensitivity of autonomic symptoms to a hypoglycemic stress (38).

5

Acute hyperglycemia

Severe hyperglycemia is associated with several neurological complications. These may arise in the setting of diabetic ketoacidosis (DKA), a feature of type 1 diabetes or nonketotic hyperosmolar syndrome usually seen in older patients. An acute painful sensory polyneuropathy specifically linked to severe hyperglycemia is also described.

DIABETIC KETOACIDOSIS

KEY POINTS

- Defined as hyperglycemia [>13.8 mmol/L (250 mg%)], ketosis and acidemia [venous pH < 7.3 or bicarbonate < 18 mmol/L (18 mEq/L)] and an anion gap (>10); usually, but not always occurs in type 1 diabetes mellitus; mortality rate 0.15% to 0.31%
- Precipitated by infection, myocardial infarction, pancreatits, appendicitis, pneumonia, medications (thiazides, glucocorticoids, sympathomimetics, some antipsychotics, others) in the setting of loss of insulin secretion
  - ○ Decreased level of consciousness (LOC) at presentation
  - ○ Cerebral edema can occur during correction (more common in children): headache, papilledema, sixth nerve palsies, confusion and decreased LOC: associated with overhydration, rapid correction, hypophosphatemia; may require mannitol
  - ○ Patients can have secondary complications including cerebral infarction, limb ischemia, myocardial infarction, arrhythmias (especially secondary to hypokalemia)
  - ○ May need to exclude an associated CNS infection or other disorder that is clouded by the neurological features of DKA

DKA is a medical emergency that may resemble a neurological problem in its presentation. A common scenario is a decline in appetite over several days with or without a flu-like illness followed by anorexia and lethargy. In response, the patient may reduce their dosing of insulin. There may be vague abdominal pain, excessive thirst and polyuria. DKA is far more common in type 1 diabetes than type 2 and more common in children. Patients exhibit hyperventilation (Kussmaul's respiration) and a fruity breath odor. It may be a presenting feature of type 1 diabetes mellitus. Severe cases may present with frank coma. Greater than 10% fluid loss may be associated with hypotension. Usually the patient improves with rehydration and insulin therapy. Acidosis and hypokalemia are frequent complications. 'Pseudohyponatremia' is a rare finding in patients with glucose levels >50 mmol/L.

Since DKA can complicate other forms of systemic illness, especially infections, it is important to be vigilant about concurrent neurological disease. Patients with decreased LOC, neck stiffness, fever, and elevated WBCs need to have meningitis excluded. DKA can also be associated with apparent worsening of preexisting neurological disease such as MS. Severe associated hypokalemia can lead to muscle paralysis and muscle necrosis from rhabdomyolysis. Hyperkalemia may complicate cerebral edema.

Cerebral edema may complicate DKA, usually 4 to 12 hours after the onset of treatment. Patients typically may have a decline in their LOC despite an initial stabilization or improvement. All of the features of raised intracranial pressure can develop: transient obscurations of vision, headache, papilledema, bilateral sixth nerve palsies and coma.

- Reference (39)

NONKETOTIC HYPEROSMOLAR SYNDROME

KEY POINTS

- Defined as glucose >33 mmol/L (600 mg%) and plasma osmolarilty >320 mOsm/L without acidosis and generally without significant ketonemia; lesser degrees of hyperglycemia also described.
- Lethargy over a few days, dehydration with thirst and polyuria, decreased LOC including coma, focal neurological signs, chorea and focal seizures with motor (tonic or clonic limbs) and visual (abnormal visual phenomena) features.
- Patients may appear volume depleted.
- Patients can develop secondary cerebral edema, rhabdomyolysis, myocardial infarction, cerebral infarction.
- Management involves rehydration, electrolyte correction, insulin therapy and correction of the underlying precipitant (see comments about "pseudohyponatremia" in DKA above).

Nonketotic hyperglycemia may develop spontaneously or following infection, pancreatitis, glucocorticoid use, cardiovascular events, dialysis or trauma.

Other causes include bowel obstruction, burns, endocrine disturbance and medications. Patients may note polyuria, polydipsia, increased thirst, fatigue, and generalized weakness. Focal neurological signs include hemiplegia, aphasia, brainstem signs, and dystonia. Seizures are most often focal (originating in a single part of the brain) and can be tonic, movement-induced or continuous (epilepsia partialis continua). Occipital lobe (visual) focal seizures are also described and can include hemianopsia (field deficit), visual hallucinations, flickering or flashing visual phenomena. Other uncommon neurological features include hallucinations, tonic eye deviation, nystagmus, abnormal pupils and meningeal signs. Patients may appear volume depleted with postural hypotension, tachycardia and dry mucous membranes. Imaging studies (MR) are usually normal or show transient changes. Treatment includes restoration of blood volume with saline, administration of insulin, avoiding overly rapid drop of serum osmolality [e.g., hold insulin when glucose is lowered to 14 mmol/L (250 mg%)], treatment of hypokalemia (risk of rhabdomyolysis). Over rapid correction of hyperosmolality may predispose patient to cerebral edema, but this is rare in nonketotic hyperglycemia. Correction of hyperglycemia may be more effective in acute seizure control than antiepileptic agents.

- References (39–41)

SUBACUTE HYPERGLYCEMIC NEUROPATHY

KEY POINTS

- Painful sensory neuropathy associated with onset of hyperglycemia or deterioration in control
- More rapid onset but less common and may be prominent in children
- Reversible, or may progress into chronic sensory motor polyneuropathy
- Buildup of uncomfortable sensory symptoms over weeks
- Burning lower limb pain, paraesthesiae and allodynia, worse at night
- May be associated with depression, weight loss and erectile dysfunction
- Resolution over a year
- Minimal physical findings of polyneuropathy and electrophysiological studies may be near normal

Subacute hyperglycemic neuropathy is not well described or differentiated from diabetic polyneuropathy, considered in chapter 9. Some authors describe this is a painful exclusively sensory, largely distal lower limb polyneuropathy with relatively few objective abnormalities. It may be reversible with correction of hyperglycemia.

- References (42–44)

6

Hypoglycemia

Hypoglycemia is a medical emergency that may mimic other neurological conditions. When suspected, presumptive therapy should be administered. Severe untreated hypoglycemia can render permanent neurological damage.

KEY POINTS

- Hypoglycemia is defined as a serum glucose level below 2.7 mmol/L (50 mg/dL).
- Assume all insulin-using diabetics have at least occasional hypoglycemia; in an emergency, assume hypoglycemia is present until proven otherwise.
- More common in type 1 (up to 40%) than type 2 diabetes mellitus (DM), but increases in type 2 diabetics who receive insulin.
- Patient may exhibit premonitory symptoms of sweating, fatigue, light-headedness, palpitations, sweating, tremor, and dizziness unless patient has autonomic neuropathy or is taking β-blocker medication that masks these symptoms.
- Diabetic patients may have hypoglycemic unawareness.
- May present with confusion, decreased level of consciousness (LOC), seizures, focal neurological signs.
- If hypoglycemia is associated with decreased LOC, seizures, or coma, treatment is a bolus of 25 to 50 mL of 50% glucose IV; 1.0-mg Glucagon SQ, IM or IV

Hypoglycemia is defined as a plasma glucose concentration below 2.7 mmol/L (50 mg/dL). Cognitive function declines below this level although patients with a history of hypoglycemia may be more resistant. Symptoms of hypoglycemia, related to rises in counterregulatory hormones, may begin at higher levels (4.0 mmol/L, 70 mg/dL). Patients with chronic hyperglycemia may experience symptoms of hypoglycemia at yet higher glucose levels. Since cognitive dysfunction can occur at glucose levels less than 2.7 mmol/L

(50 mg/dL) and glucagon levels (to counteract declines in glucose) fail to rise, patients may be unaware, become seriously impaired, and may fail to take adequate protective measures. Driving performance is impaired at glucose levels less than 3.8 mmol/L (68 mg/dL). Recurrent hypoglycemia may also contribute to an increased risk of hypoglycemic unawareness because control of hypoglycemia restores sensitivity of autonomic symptoms to hypoglycemic stress.

CLINICAL FEATURES

- *Symptoms of early hypoglycemia:* anxiety, tachycardia, palpitations, cold perspiration, nausea, dizziness, and tremor; these may be absent in a patient with autonomic neuropathy or if β-adrenergic blocking agents are being taken. There may be hunger and headache. Symptoms may be prominent in the mornings or after prolonged intervals without meals. Hypoglycemia may precipitate a migraine attack.
- *Cognitive symptoms:* decreased attention and concentration, drowsiness, poor memory, disorientation, bizarre behavior, change in speech, clumsiness, tremor (cognitive symptoms can take up to an hour to recover after correction of hypoglycemia).
- *Seizures:* generalized tonic-clonic, status epilepticus, focal or multifocal.
- *Focal signs (less common):* transient hemiplegia (alternating sides), other TIA-like symptoms, choreiform or athetoid movements.
- *Clues to nocturnal hypoglycemia:* vivid dreams, morning headaches, chronic fatigue, poor sleep and depression; death during sleep may occur in young type 1 diabetic patients secondary to a hypoglycemia-induced arrhythmia.
- Failure to awaken despite correction of glucose levels may be secondary to ongoing nonconvulsive seizures (urgent EEG indicated) or from severe neuronal damage secondary to hypoglycemia (diffuse cortical, basal ganglia, dentate gyrus involvement).
- Severe hypoglycemia is associated with coma and seizures; some instances result in permanent neurological impairment or persistent vegetative state.

CAUSES OF HYPOGLYCEMIA

- Insulin overdose (intentional or nonintentional)
- Prolonged action of oral sulfonylureas, especially in elderly patients
- Hepatic disease and ethanol abuse
- Insulinoma and IGF-secreting tumors (sarcoma, mesothelioma, and hepatoma)
- Other endocrine disorders: pituitary lesions, adrenal insufficiency (rare)
- Other medical conditions: renal disease, sepsis
- Malnutrition (usually only mild)

- Drugs: acetaminophen, ASA, amphetamines, chloramphenicol, haloperidol, MAO inhibitors, phenothiazines, sulfa drugs, pentamidine, manganese, others
- In diabetic patients: early type 1 remission, postpartum, renal impairment, exercise, change in insulin regimen or injection site, change in lifestyle, dieting, breast-feeding, malabsorption or GI disease, gastroparesis, endocrine failure, medication error, deliberate overdosing, other

TREATMENT

- Oral therapy if conscious (15 g for mild, 20 g for severe, e.g., 4 teaspoonfuls of sugar dissolved in water)
- Absorption of rectal glucose is unreliable and not recommended
- Glucagon 1.0-mg SQ, IM or IV (onset of action 8–10 minutes, IM, 1 minute IV) (vials are 1 mg/1 mL)
- Bolus of 25 to 50 g of 50% glucose IV (20% glucose may cause less venous irritation)
- Recurrent hypoglycemia can occur after initial treatment—vigilance is required
- References (38,40,45)

7

Cerebrovascular disease

Diabetic persons are at significant risk of developing cerebrovascular disease. "Stroke" is a broad term for these complications and includes both cerebral infarction and hemorrhage. Transient ischemic attacks (TIAs) can identify patients at risk for subsequent cerebral infarction.

KEY POINTS

- Stroke is a neurovascular syndrome.
- Diabetes is a risk factor for stroke, particularly ischemic stroke.
- Hyperglycemia is a poor prognostic factor following ischemic stroke. It remains unclear if treatment of hyperglycemia in the acute phase is useful.

DEFINITIONS

- Stroke is a syndrome of sudden neurologic symptoms caused by vascular pathology in the brain or in the vessels leading to or from the brain.
- Stroke is divided into types with associated frequency.
  - i. Ischemia (blocked artery—lack of blood flow) ~85% of all stroke
    - ○ Ischemic stroke
    - ○ TIA
  - ii. Hemorrhage (ruptured artery or vein—bleeding) ~15% of all stroke
    - ○ Intracerebral hemorrhage (ICH)
    - ○ Subarachnoid hemorrhage (SAH)
  - iii. Venous sinus or cortical vein thrombosis—<1% of all stroke

CLINICAL FEATURES

- Stroke is sudden and maximal at onset.
- Symptoms are determined by brain location.
- Common symptoms are as follows:
  - ○ Motor—weakness, paralysis on one side of the body—face, arm, leg
  - ○ Aphasia—language disturbance (verbal, reading, writing)

- ○ Hemispatial neglect—right hemisphere syndrome of inattention
- ○ Vision loss—hemifield or quadrantic field visual loss
- Other symptoms include the following:
  - ○ Sensory loss—anesthesia or paresthesia on one side of the body
  - ○ Ataxia of limbs, ataxia of gait
  - ○ Diplopia
  - ○ Dysphagia, dysarthria
  - ○ Altered level of consciousness (LOC)
  - ○ Apnea
- General symptoms include the following:
  - ○ Headache—sudden, thunderclap, "worst headache of my life" is typically associated with SAH or venous sinus thrombosis, but is also seen with acute ischemic stroke and ICH
  - ○ Vomiting
  - ○ Diaphoresis
  - ○ Tachycardia—particularly with acute onset atrial fibrillation
  - ○ Hypertension—very common in the acute period (first 48 hours)

DIAGNOSIS

- Diagnosis is based on clinical signs and symptoms.
- Statistically, acute neurological deficits in an adult are a stroke until proven otherwise.
- Imaging (CT or MR) is required to distinguish ischemia from hemorrhage; statistically, ischemia is a more likely cause of an acute neurological syndrome, but reliable rules for clinical prediction to distinguish hemorrhage from ischemia are not available (Fig. 7.1).
- Acute angiographic imaging (CTA or MRA) is critical in acute decision making.
- The majority (~70%) of ischemic stroke syndromes are minor or mild, such patients are not eligible for thrombolysis.

CAUSES

- Ischemic stroke (cerebral infarction or "infarcts") is divided into subtypes by mechanism.
- TIA has the same causes as ischemic stroke but TIA is transient (by definition lasts < 24 hours).

Large Artery Disease

- Carotid artery atherosclerotic disease—carotid artery plaque with associated plaque rupture, thrombus formation on the plaque resulting in arteroembolic stroke

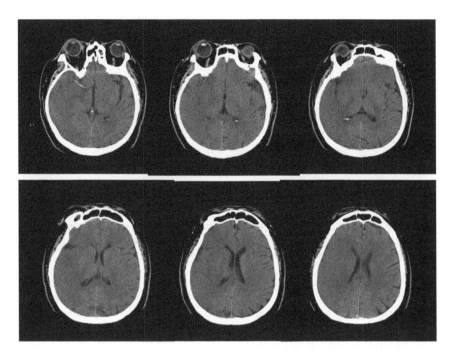

Figure 7.1 An example of unenhanced CT brain scan findings in a patient with a large middle cerebral artery territory infarction (stroke). Note that the right hemisphere (*left side of the picture*) has extensive hypodensity (*darker*) in each of the CT slices shown. Unlike the normal side, there is loss of the normal cortical delineation of gray and white matter in all slices shown and there is early swelling with some compression of the right lateral ventricle by mass effect.

- Vertebral artery atherosclerotic disease—vertebrobasilar artery plaque with associated plaque rupture, thrombus formation on the plaque resulting in arteroembolic stroke
- Intracranial atherosclerotic disease—plaque with associated plaque rupture, thrombus formation on the plaque resulting in arteroembolic stroke (Fig. 7.2)

Cardioembolic

- Atrial fibrillation—typically a thrombus forms in the left atrial appendage then embolises
- Mural thrombus postmyocardial infarction or cardiomyopathy
- Valvular heart disease
- Endocarditis—infectious or marantic
- Aortic arch disease—considered cardioembolic, but the mechanism is otherwise similar to large artery disease
- Paradoxical embolus through an atrial connection, such as a PFO (persistent foramen ovale) or ventricular septal defect

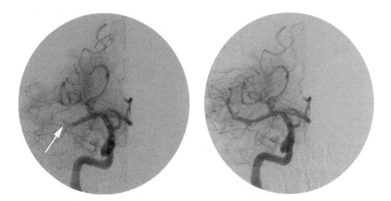

Figure 7.2 Occlusion of the right middle cerebral artery (*arrow*) demonstrated by a cerebral angiogram study. Note the recanalization of the proximal right middle cerebral artery with intra-arterial tPA in the right hand panel.

- Congenital heart disease
- Embolism to the brain is more common than embolism to the splanchnic bed or legs because of the high proportion of blood flow that normally goes to the brain; laminar flow of blood in the aorta also predisposes the transport of emboli to the brain

Lacunar

- Small-vessel (microvascular) disease—mechanism of occlusion is not fully understood. Arteroembolic and cardioembolic mechanisms occur but are likely less common than intrinsic small artery disease. These small arteries may have microatheroma with associated plaque rupture or undergo lipohyalinosis and degenerate with luminal collapse resulting in ischemia. Distinguishing mechanisms for lacunar stroke may be clinically impossible in individual patients (Fig. 7.3).
- Diabetes and hypertension are important risk factors for lacunar stroke.

Other Known Causes

- Dissection (separation of the layers of the vascular wall by blood)
- Accelerated atherosclerosis in arteries exposed to previous radiation (e.g., carotid artery after head and neck irradiation for tumor)
- Vasculitis
  - Infectious (e.g., syphilis, aspergillus)
  - Autoimmune
- Vasculopathy
  - Reversible segmental vasospasm
  - Drug-induced vasospasm (e.g., cocaine, decongestant nasal sprays, crystal methamphetamine, dietary weight loss supplements)

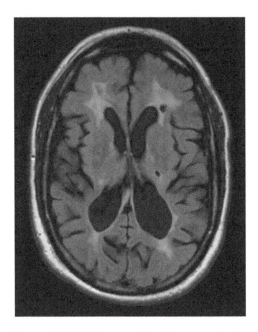

Figure 7.3 MR images (FLAIR sequence) from a patient with diabetes-related white matter disease and lacunar lesions evident in the left hemisphere (*right side of picture*). There are also white matter hyperintensity changes around the ventricles.

- Hypercoagulable states
  - Cancer
  - Antiphospholipid antibody syndrome
- Cryptogenic or unknown
- Clear cause not identified despite complete workup

Subarachnoid Hemorrhage

- The commonest cause of SAH is trauma; otherwise "SAH" refers to an atraumatic cause
- Atraumatic SAH is typically caused by rupture of an intracranial aneurysm
  - Berry/saccular aneurysms (increased risk of rupture if size > 5–10 mm)
  - Fusiform nonsaccular aneurysms are less common
  - Arteriovenous malformations
  - Rare causes include dissecting aneurysms, mycotic aneurysms

Intracerebral Hemorrhage

- Intracerebral hemorrhage (ICH) is divided into lobar and deep types.
- Lobar hemorrhage is considered hemorrhage focused on the gray-white junction within 1 cm of the cortical surface. Lobar hemorrhage is

commonly due to amyloid angiopathy, a condition associated with Alzheimer's disease.
- Deep or subcortical hemorrhage involves the thalamus, basal ganglia, deep cerebellar nuclei, or pons. Hypertension is typically the underlying cause.

EPIDEMIOLOGY AND RISK FACTORS

Risk Factors

- Hypertension is the most important risk factor for stroke in both non-diabetic and diabetic patients
  - The largest magnitude of risk from hypertension is for ICH
  - Hypertension is an important risk factor for ischemia (TIA, infarction)
  - Hypertension is a small magnitude risk factor for SAH
- Hypercholesterolemia
  - Risk factor for atherosclerotic disease
  - Very low cholesterol may be a risk factor for ICH
- Diabetes mellitus
  - See later in text

Risk States

- Cardiac—atrial fibrillation, valvular heart disease, recent myocardial infarction (MI)
- Large artery atherosclerotic disease (see earlier text)

Special Considerations in Diabetics

- Hyperglycemia is a strong negative predictor of outcome in the acute and subacute stages after stroke—hyperglycemic patients are more likely to die, to suffer complications such as secondary ICH and to be disabled. This is true of both diabetics and nondiabetics.
- It is not known if treatment of hyperglycemia (e.g., using insulin infusions) improves stroke outcome. Trials to date are inconclusive.
- Diabetes mellitus is a negative predictor of outcome.
- Diabetics suffer a higher prevalence of ischemic stroke (cerebral infarction) compared with hemorrhagic forms of stroke.
- Diabetic patients have a greater tendency to suffer lacunar stroke and show evidence of small vessel ischemic disease. This may be due to their high prevalence of comorbid hypertension.
- The high prevalence of white matter disease/small-vessel ischemic disease among diabetic patients has implications for cognitive impairment and dementia (see chap. 14).
- It remains unclear if aggressive, normoglycemic treatment reduces the long-term risk of stroke.

- Aggressive treatment to achieve normoglycemia reduces retinal disease, neuropathy, and nephropathy. The evidence that it reduces macrovascular complications of diabetes (coronary artery disease, stroke) remains limited.
- Long-term follow-up of the DCCT and United Kingdom Prospective Diabetes Study (UKPDS) studies suggests that a "legacy effect" of early aggressive treatment may exist. Early, aggressive treatment of patients may result in a long-term (>10 year) reduction of macrovascular complications. Aggressive treatment of patients with well-established diabetes mellitus may paradoxically result in worse outcomes and increased death.

PROGNOSIS

- Stroke outcome is largely determined by initial stroke severity.
- Death is additionally predicted by age at stroke onset and comorbid illness.
- Other factors such as baseline clinical risk factors, gender, and treatment have an overall moderate effect on stroke outcome.

TREATMENT

Acute

- Hyperacute stroke in diabetics is treated the same as in nondiabetics.
- Thrombolysis is offered according to usual criteria.
- While there is no randomized evidence that treatment of hyperglycemia is useful, many physicians will routinely treat glucose > 12 mM (216 mg%) with short-acting insulin.
- Diabetic patients are more prone to infectious complications of stroke (see chap. 15); careful stroke unit care is warranted to prevent these complications.

Prevention

- Prevention should be designed to treat both (*i*) risk states and (*ii*) risk factors.
- Search for cardioembolic source such as atrial fibrillation—initiate anticoagulation if required.
- Search for large artery disease such as extracranial internal carotid artery stenosis—initiate carotid revascularization (endarterectomy or stent) if appropriate.
- Most important risk factor to treat is hypertension.
  - Aggressive approach is warranted—target average systolic blood pressure (SBP) < 130 mmHg.
- Treat cholesterol.
  - Aggressive approach is warranted—the target LDL-C (low-density lipoprotein cholesterol level) is < 2.0 mM (77 mg%).

- Discontinue smoking.
- Treat overweight, abdominal obesity, metabolic syndrome with weight loss, exercise, and diet.
- Treat diabetes mellitus.
  ○ In well-established diabetes mellitus, it is likely not true that aggressive management of hyperglycemia will result in reduction in stroke risk.
  ○ In new-onset diabetes mellitus, aggressive management of hyperglycemia may result in long-term reduction in the risk of macrovascular complications (so-called "legacy effect").
- Use antiplatelet agents.
  ○ ASA alone is usually adequate (low-dose ASA)—any dose between 75–325 mg is acceptable (81 mg routinely used in Canada; coated preparations preferable).
  ○ Clopidogrel or combination ASA plus slow-release dipyridamole are also effective.
  ○ Be aware of drug interactions in treatment choices (e.g., clopidogrel and proton pump inhibitors used for GI disease).
  ○ There is no evidence that long-term double antiplatelet therapy with ASA plus clopidogrel prevents stroke. The MATCH study suggests that an increased risk of hemorrhage outweighs any benefit in reduction of ischemic events.
- References (46–48).

8

Neuropathic pain

Neuropathic pain is often a difficult and intractable problem in diabetic persons. It appears in both type 1 and 2 diabetes mellitus, sometimes early in the course of the disease. Although primarily seen in diabetes clinics or general practice, patients with painful diabetic polyneuropathy (DPN) may seek treatment from neurologists, pain specialists, anesthesiologists, and others.

KEY POINTS

- Pain in patients with neurological disease is not necessarily "neuropathic" — investigate other causes.
- The definition of "neuropathic pain" was originally limited to pain from disease or damage to peripheral nerves.
- Key descriptors of neuropathic pain include tingling, prickling, "pins and needles," lancinating or shooting sensations, electrical sensations (including electrical shocks), and burning. Patients may also use less specific terms such as tight, squeezing, aching, crushing, throbbing, knife-like, and swelling. The pain should be localized to the territory of a peripheral nerve, nerve root, for example, dermatomal or stocking and glove.
- Neuropathic pain is found in 7% to 20% of diabetic subjects (42).
- Allodynia refers to pain caused by a sensory stimulus that is ordinarily innocuous such as touch, mild pinprick, and cold.
- Some patients with polyneuropathy may have neuropathic pain with no objective findings on examination.
- Step therapy starting with simple analgesics is appropriate followed by antiepileptic agents (gabapentin, pregabalin), serotonin/norepinephrine uptake inhibitors (antidepressants), and opioids in some instances.

A new neurological definition of neuropathic pain has been published (49): "Pain arising as a direct consequence of a lesion or disease affecting the somatosensory system" graded as follows: (*i*) pain with a distinct neuroanatomically plausible distribution; (*ii*) a history suggestive of a relevant lesion or disease affecting the peripheral or central somatosensory system; (*iii*) demonstration of the distinct neuroanatomically plausible distribution by at least one confirmatory test; and (*iv*) demonstration of the relevant lesion or disease by at least one confirmatory test. This is broader than the original concept in that "neuropathic" refers to pain arising from central or peripheral neurons. The descriptors for pain arising from the central nervous system may differ from those arising from peripheral nerve damage. From peripheral damage, symptoms are described as tingling, prickling, "pins and needles," lancinating or shooting, electrical, burning, walking on stones or burning sand. Neuropathic pain in diabetes can be disabling leading to inability to work, reduced quality of life, and depression.

CLINICAL DIAGNOSIS

- Full neurological assessment is often necessary to confirm the cause.
- Perform MR imaging of lumbar intraspinal space if associated lumbar pain is present.
- Perform electrophysiological tests (EMG, nerve conduction) if the findings are atypical for DPN.

Differential Diagnosis of Pain Syndromes

Stocking and Glove Neuropathic Pain

- DPN
- Other forms of polyneuropathy: nutritional/ethanol related (e.g., thiamine deficiency); inflammatory [chronic inflammatory demyelinating polyneuropathy (CIDP), anti-myelin-associated glycoprotein (anti-MAG)], paraneoplastic, hypothyroid, B12 deficiency, HIV infection, neurotoxins (including chemotherapy), many others
- "Pseudoneuropathy"—a combination of lumbar spinal stenosis and bilateral carpal tunnel syndrome
- Stocking and glove tingling syndrome secondary to foramen magnum lesions (compressive or intrinsic lesions)

Arm or Hand Neuropathic Pain

- Entrapment neuropathy
- Mononeuritis multiplex
- Radiculopathy
- Herpes zoster
- Brachial neuritis
- Brachial plexus infiltration or compression
- Cervical cord lesion

Leg or Foot Neuropathic Pain (see chap. 3)

- DPN
- Radiculopathy (single, multiple, spinal stenosis)

- Mononeuritis multiplex
- Herpes zoster
- Lumbosacral plexopathy [diabetic lumbosacral plexopathy (DLSP) or other causes]
- Tabes dorsalis
- Lumbar or sacral cord lesion

Truncal Neuropathic Pain

- Thoracic intercostal or abdominal radicular (truncal) neuropathy
- Herpes zoster
- Radiculopathy secondary to intraspinal compressive lesion
- Thoracic cord lesion

THERAPY[a]

General Measures

- Exclude other causes of pain (see earlier).
- Evaluate for concurrent depression.
- Improve glycemic control, treat hypertension, obesity, hyperlipidemia, smoking.
- May be exacerbated by soft tissue injuries, ulcers.
- Use a blanket cradle to lift bedclothes from the feet and reduce allodynia.

Antiepileptic Agents

α2 δ1 Subunit Inhibitors

- Gabapentin; initial dose 300 mg q.h.s. then titrate to 300 mg t.i.d. (maximum 4000 mg daily); dizziness, fatigue, and cognitive complaints with initial doses or higher doses; renal excretion, reduce dose in renal failure; leg edema
- Pregabalin; initial dose 75 mg q.h.s. then titrate to 150 mg b.i.d. (maximum 600 mg daily); dizziness, fatigue, and cognitive complaints; overall adverse effects similar to gabapentin; reduce dose in renal failure

Older Antiepileptics

- Phenytoin; 300 mg once daily, begin with full dose; check levels; side effects: ataxia and nystagmus with high levels, osteoporosis, gum

---

[a]Therapeutic agents are only briefly described here and recommendations are listed as suggestions only. Clinicians should be aware that recommended therapy for pain or other disorders may change with time and the regimens and approvals vary with the jurisdiction. All therapeutics should be used only with complete references to indications, contraindications, adverse effects, and dosage. These suggestions are also not based on specific FDA approval.

hypertrophy, liver function abnormalities, rash; long-term therapy can cause sensory polyneuropathy

- Carbamazepine; 400 to 1200 mg daily, titrate up slowly; chewtabs may be helpful on a p.r.n. basis; more helpful in patients with lancinating, neuralgic, electrical pain; avoid if ECG shows heart block; other side effects: dizziness, rash
- Topiramate; start at 25 mg twice daily and titrate up (maximum 400 mg/day); side effects: somnolence, dizziness, ataxia, speech disturbance, fatigue, cognitive side effects, paresthesia; *weight loss* (a helpful side effect for type 2 diabetic patients)
- Lamotrigine; start at 25 mg daily or lower; titrate slowly to a maximum dose of 150 to 250 mg twice daily; risk of serious rash (including Stevens–Johnson syndrome), interactions with other antiepileptic medications; side effects: dizziness, somnolence, headache, diplopia, ataxia, nausea, asthenia

Serotonin and Norepinephrine Uptake Inhibitors (SSRIs and SSNRIs; Antidepressants)

Newer SSNRIs

- Venlafaxine start at 37.5 mg/day; increase weekly by 37.5 mg/day to 150 to 225 mg/day; side effects: nausea, dizziness, drowsiness, hyperhidrosis, hypertension, constipation
- Duloxetine 30 to 60 mg daily; risk of hepatotoxicity; side effects: nausea, dry mouth, constipation, somnolence, hyperhidrosis, and decreased appetite

Older SSNRIs

- Amitriptyline; start 10 to 25 mg q.h.s. once daily then titrate up to 100 to 150 mg; side effects: next day drowsiness, lethargy, dry mouth, constipation, bladder retention; may help with prominent nocturnal pain; use with caution in patients with cardiac conduction abnormalities; contraindicated in glaucoma or patients taking MAO inhibitors
- Nortryptyline, imipramine; similar dosing, side effects as with amitriptyline but slightly less sedation

Opioids

- Tramadol 37.5 mg p.o. q3-6h, often combined with 325 mg of acetaminophen [long-acting preparations starting at 100–150 mg daily (once daily) to a maximum of 300–400 mg daily]; opioid side effects include cognitive dysfunction, somnolence, respiratory depression, constipation, pruritis, dizziness, nausea, vomiting; risk of addiction and withdrawal syndrome
- Long-acting (controlled release) oxycodone 10 to 100 mg divided into twice daily administration (ratio of efficacy to morphine is 1.5 mg

oxycodone/1.0 mg morphine); opioid side effects include cognitive dysfunction, somnolence, respiratory depression, constipation, pruritis, dizziness, nausea, vomiting, dry mouth, headache; risk of addiction and withdrawal syndrome
- Morphine 30 to 60 mg b.i.d. of long-acting preparation (e.g., MS Contin); may be the treatment of choice with severe unremittant pain and severe underlying systemic disease (e.g., renal failure, cardiac disease); side effects: cognitive dysfunction including hallucinations, somnolence, respiratory depression, constipation, pruritis, dizziness, nausea, vomiting; addiction risk and withdrawal syndrome

Combinations

- Gabapentin and morphine provide synergistic pain control allowing individual agents to be used at lower doses (50,51).

Topical Agents

- Lidocaine patch (5%), capsaicin with or without menthol

Other Approaches

- Isorbide dinitrate spray, mexiletine, dextromethorphan, memantine, cannabinoids (nabilone, others)

PAIN SCALES

- Pain scales are designed to rate the efficacy of analgesics in clinical practice. They are most frequently used in clinical trials of pain therapies. Often pain severity is graded from 0 (no pain) to 10 (severe pain). Formal examples of pain scales include the McGill Pain Questionnaire (52), the Visual Analogue Scale (53), and the Brief Pain Inventory (54).
- References (42,55,56).

9

Polyneuropathy

Diabetic polyneuropathy (DPN) is among the most common complications of diabetes mellitus. It should not be viewed as an "end-stage" complication of diabetes since it may occur in children, or soon after the diagnosis of diabetes mellitus.

KEY POINTS

- DPN may be observed in approximately 50% of type 1 or type 2 diabetics using rigorous diagnostic techniques.
- Symptomatic neuropathy occurs in approximately 20% of diabetics (57).
- Most common early symptoms are positive sensory symptoms-tingling, prickling, paresthesiae, "pins and needles" in the distal toes (longest nerves first targeted) or pain in a "stocking and glove" distribution.
- Classical features are stocking and glove distribution symptoms (pain, numbness, tingling) with or without sensory loss.
- Early sensory polyneuropathy (including painful polyneuropathy) has been linked to impaired fasting glucose (IFG) or impaired glucose tolerance (IGT).
- Autonomic involvement may accompany early polyneuropathy.
- Motor involvement usually occurs later and involves distal muscles.
- DPN is often accompanied by superimposed entrapment neuropathies, autonomic involvement.
- DPN is a major risk factor for lower extremity ulceration: regular foot inspection is essential.
- Other causes of polyneuropathy should be excluded: B_{12} deficiency, hypothyroidism, HIV infection and treatment, underlying neoplasm, other nutritional deficiencies, ethanol use, others.

CLINICAL FEATURES

Polyneuropathy (DPN, diabetic polyneuropathy) secondary to diabetes is the most common form of neuropathy worldwide. DPN usually presents with spontaneous positive (paresthesiae described as prickling, tingling, "pins and needles," burning, lancinating, jabbing, electrical shocks, crawling, itching, "tightness," abnormal sensation to temperature, pain) or negative (numbness, injury insensitivity) sensory symptoms in the distal toes. Over time, symptoms may advance up the foot and leg to involve the fingers and hands. Neuropathic pain may be prominent and early despite minimal signs of polyneuropathy, and it may lead to sleep deprivation. There may be muscle cramps. Allodynia is the sensation of pain from normally nonpainful stimuli such as bed covers or walking. Walking may be painful and hesitant or unsteady and falls may result. Some patients present with foot ulcers.

One of the more interesting and comprehensive papers written on the subject was by Rundles in 1945 (58) describing a series of 125 patients:

> *Numbness, tingling and paresthesiae such as "cold" feelings, aching and burning pains, and so forth, were usually prominent among the patient's complaints. Severe "shooting pains" both in deep and in superficial tissues were noted in more than one-fourth of the patients. The cramps, aches, and pains were characteristically worse upon exposure to cold and at night. The touch of bedclothes was often unbearable, sleep and rest impossible. Morphine and codeine were frequently necessary over periods of weeks or months to relieve pain. Patients so afflicted often became mentally depressed and emotionally unstable after a time . . ."*

There is loss of light touch with either reduced or absent sensation (hypesthesia and analgesia, respectively). Light touch sensation is assessed by a cotton piece or light brush, pinprick by using new safety pins (analgesia is defined by an inability of the patient to distinguish the sharp from blunt end of a pin), cold sensation by using a cooled tuning fork (or other approaches), vibration sensation by using a 128 or 256 tuning fork, and proprioception by testing sensation to movement of the distal phalanx of the large toe. Sensory loss may involve only the distal toes but may also extend to the ankle or further up the legs and thighs. The loss is described as "length dependent" because the longest fibers supplying the feet are involved first. With moderate or advanced neuropathy, sensory loss is described as "stocking and glove" because of the disappearance of distal axon branches. There may be loss of ankle reflexes earlier and of the knee reflexes or upper limb deep tendon reflexes later (Fig. 9.1). Early motor changes are atrophy of the extensor digitorum brevis (EDB) muscle but weakness of toe and foot dorsiflexors occurs later. There may be clawing of the toes. Foot atrophy and abnormalities of posture contribute to foot ulceration and gait imbalance. Loss of distal autonomic fibers results in loss of sweating in the extremity causing dry skin that is more easily cracked, damaged, and infected.

Polyneuropathy is sometimes divided into subtypes, although substantial overlap exists:

1. Predominantly sensory
   "Small fiber"-pain, loss of pinprick and thermal sensation, preservation of reflexes, loss of epidermal axons; nerve conduction may be normal

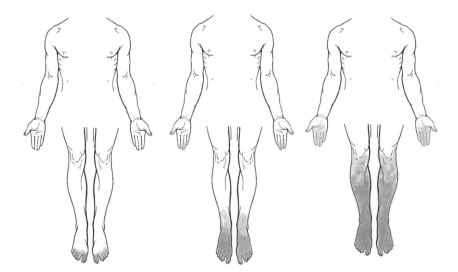

Figure 9.1 Illustration of progressive stocking and glove changes typical of diabetic polyneuropathy. Both symptoms, such as pain and paresthesiae (tingling) and signs, such as sensory loss involve the toes followed by the proximal foot and fingers as the disorder progresses.

> "Large fiber"-ataxia (unsteadiness), loss of deep tendon reflexes, loss of light touch, vibration perception, prominent sensory nerve conduction changes
> "Mixed" large and small fiber
2. Painful sensory
> "Chronic painful sensory"
> "Acute polyneuropathy from hyperglycemia"—this is a painful polyneuropathy developing soon after the diagnosis or during a period of poor glycemic control. A similar version is also linked to the onset of rapid glycemic control and consequently labeled "insulin neuritis"
3. Sensorimotor (includes sensory and motor deficits)
4. Predominantly autonomic (see chap. 13)
5. Predominantly motor (controversial)
6. Combinations of the above

DIFFERENTIAL DIAGNOSIS OF DPN

Deficiency

- B vitamin deficiency (thiamine, B_{12}, multiple B vitamins)
- Vitamin E deficiency

Infectious and Inflammatory

- HIV infection
- Leprosy
- Lyme disease
- Hepatitis C
- Guillain–Barré syndrome (GBS)
- Chronic inflammatory demyelinating polyneuropathy (CIDP)
- Anti-MAG neuropathy, Lewis–Sumner syndrome, distal acquired demyelinating symmetric neuropathy (DADS)
- Neuropathies in association with monoclonal gammopathies
- Primary biliary cirrhosis

Endocrine

- Hypothyroidism
- Acromegaly (with diabetes)

Drugs and Toxins

- Antibiotics—metronidazole, isoniazid, nitrofurantoin
- Antineoplastic agents—vincristine, vinblastine, cisplatinum, others
- Ethanol (often in association with thiamine deficiency)
- Pesticides
- Pyridoxine
- Antiretroviral therapies
- Interferon-α
- Anti-TNF-α treatment for inflammatory disorders
- Sinemet (B_{12} deficiency)
- Others

Metabolic

- Hepatic cirrhosis
- Renal failure
- Critical illness (sepsis and multiorgan failure)
- Acquired amyloidosis
- Gastric surgery

Congenital/Inherited

- Charcot–Marie–Tooth diseases (CMTs)—multiple subtypes
- Inherited sensitivity to pressure palsy (HSPP)
- Inherited amyloidosis
- Hereditary sensory and autonomic neuropathies

Vascular

- Necrotizing vasculitis (confined to peripheral nerves or in association with systemic vasculitis)
- Severe peripheral vascular disease
- Cryoglobulinemia (with or without hepatitis C)

Neoplastic

- Paraneoplastic neuropathies (anti-Hu, Ma, others)
- Leptomeningeal carcinomatosis, lymphomatosis, gliomatosis
- Angioendotheliosis
- Primary intraneural lympoma

DISTINGUISHING DPN FROM CIDP

- This is important because chronic inflammatory demyelinating polyneuropathy (CIDP) may respond to immunomodulatory therapy (prednisone, IVIG, plasma exchange).
- CIDP is a subacute progressive or relapsing neuropathy, usually involving motor fibers and rendering prominent weakness.
- Electrophysiological studies identify striking features of primary demyelination: prolonged distal motor latencies, slowed conduction velocities, temporal dispersion of CMAP responses, and conduction block in motor fibers.
- Nerve biopsy identifies primary demyelination.

  CIDP is an immune-mediated neuropathy with predominant demyelination and a slowly progressive or, stepwise largely motor course that can occur in diabetic or nondiabetic subjects. It is distinguished by having more prominent motor involvement with electrophysiological features of demyelination. Prednisone, intravenous γ-globulin or plasma exchange are effective treatments.

OTHER DIAGNOSTIC TECHNIQUES (SEE CHAP. 2)

- The Semmes–Weinstein 10 g monofilament is pressed against the dorsum of the large toe until it bends and the patient, with eyes closed, is asked to identify when the stimuli are applied (e.g., 5 times on each toe). Plantar application has also been described. As a test of mechanical sensitivity, this test predicts the risk of foot ulceration with yearly screening (43,59).
- Nerve conduction and EMG: The earliest changes in DPN are declines in the amplitude of the sural SNAP, sural sensory conduction velocity slowing, and peroneal motor conduction slowing. In severe neuropathy, there may be widespread loss of SNAPs, diffuse mild-moderate conduction velocity slowing, and distal denervation by needle EMG with enlarged remodeled motor unit potentials indicative of denervation with reinnervation (Table 9.1). Prominent features of primary demyelination (temporal

Table 9.1 Grading Scales for the Severity of Polyneuropathy

(a) San Antonio criteria for the diagnosis of diabetic polyneuropathy
Class I polyneuropathy without signs or symptoms
A—Abnormal autonomic testing, QST or neither
B—Abnormal nerve conduction, or autonomic testing and QST
C—Abnormal nerve conduction and autonomic testing or QST or both abnormal
Class II polyneuropathy with signs or symptoms (or both)
A—Symptoms, no signs, autonomic, and QST studies may or may not be abnormal
B—Signs with or without symptoms and nerve conduction or autonomic and QST abnormal
C—One or both of symptoms and signs and nerve conduction and autonomic testing or
    QST or both abnormal

(b) Modified Toronto Neuropathy Scale

Symptom scores (0 = absent, 1 = present but does not interfere with well-being or daily
    living, 2 = present, interferes with well-being but not daily living, 3 = present and
    interferes with well-being and daily living): scored for each of foot pain, numbness,
    tingling, weakness, ataxia, upper limb symptoms
Sensory test scores (0 = normal, 1 = reduced at toes only, 2 = reduced beyond the toes
    as far as ankles only, 3 = reduced above the ankles and/or absent at the toes): scored for
    each of pinprick, temperature, light touch, vibration, position sense
Maximum score = 33 (0 = normal)

(c) Utah Neuropathy Scale

Motor examination (left and right): Normal (0) or weak (2) great toe extension. Total =
    out of 4
Pin sensation (left and right): Normal (0), or for each segment of reduced sensation
    (1 point for each of toes, foot, lower leg, mid leg, upper leg to knee), or for each
    segment of absent sensation (2 points for each of toes, foot, lower leg, mid leg, upper
    leg to knee). Total = out of 24
Allodynia/hyperesthesia (left and right): Normal (0), or if present in toes or foot (1).
    Total = out of 2
Large fiber sensation (left and right): Normal (0), or diminished (1), or absent (2) for
    each of great toe vibration, great toe joint position (vibration sensation duration also
    timed). Total = out of 8
Deep tendon reflex at ankle (left and right): Normal (0), or diminished (1), or absent (2).
    Total = out of 4
Total score = out of 42 (0 = normal)

(d) Michigan Neuropathy Scale

Sensory impairment (left and right): Normal (0), decreased (1) or absent (2) for vibration
    at big toe, 10 g monofilament, pinprick on dorsum of great toe
Muscle strength (left and right): Normal (0), mild to moderate weakness (1), severe
    weakness (2), absent (3) for finger spread, great toe extension, ankle dorsiflexion
Deep tendon reflexes (left and right): Present (0), present with reinforcement (1), absent
    (2) for biceps brachii, triceps brachii, quadriceps femoris (knee), achilles (ankle)
Total score = out of 46 (0 = normal)

(Continued)

Table 9.1 Grading Scales for the Severity of Polyneuropathy (*Continued*)

(e) Mayo Clinic/Dyck diabetic polyneuropathy classification

N0—No polyneuropathy

N1a—Asymptomatic polyneuropathy with abnormal nerve conduction in at least two nerves, a heart rate deep breathing abnormality or an abnormal result on a composite scale [such as the NIS plus 7 (see below), also described by Mayo/Dyck]

N1b—Fufills N1a plus an abnormality on neurological examination (QST abnormality qualifies)

N2a—Symptomatic mild DPN (less than 50% weakness of foot dorsiflexion)

N2b—Symptomatic severe DPN (more than 50% dorsiflexion weakness, unable to stand on heels)

N3—Disabling DPN (patient unable to walk because of weakness or sensory loss, disabling pain or autonomic symptoms such as incontinence, diarrhea, postural lightheadedness)

"NIS+7" score is a composite score based on an NIS and seven abnormal tests (QST, heart rate with deep breathing, 5 attributes from nerve conduction studies of the peroneal, tibial, and sural nerve). NIS is based on a 0–4 rating on a 37-point scale that involves cranial nerve function, motor function, sensation and reflexes. NIS-LL refers to a subset of the NIS scale focused on the lower limbs. See Ref. 67 for details.

Abbreviation: NIS, Neuropathy Impairment Score.
Source: (a) is from Ref. 62, (b) is from Ref. 63, (c) is from Ref. 64, (d) is from Ref. 65, (e) is from Ref. 66. Scales are summarized here with permission of the authors and publisher.

dispersion and conduction block of CMAPs) are uncommon except in severe neuropathy and at sites of nerve entrapment (Fig. 9.2).

- Computerized quantitative sensory testing (QST) uses calibrated electronic interfaces (see chap. 2) for thermal thresholds (warm, cold), heat as pain, touch pressure, and vibration. The thresholds in the feet are raised in DPN.
- Autonomic testing can include a variety of methods useful for testing for small fiber involvement (see chap. 13).
- Newer methods, not in routine clinical use to date, include skin biopsy to count epidermal axons and corneal confocal microscopy to examine corneal sensory axons (rapid, noninvasive analysis of small fibers).
- Sural nerve biopsy is not recommended for routine clinical use; it is used for the diagnosis of unusual or progressive neuropathy to identify other causes.
- CSF protein is often elevated in DPN but pleocytosis (the presence of WBCs in CSF) is not expected.

CAUSES

- The cause of DPN is controversial.
- Vascular risk factors are associated with the development of DPN, but there is no evidence that ischemia or hypoxia are responsible; it may not be a "microvascular" complication.

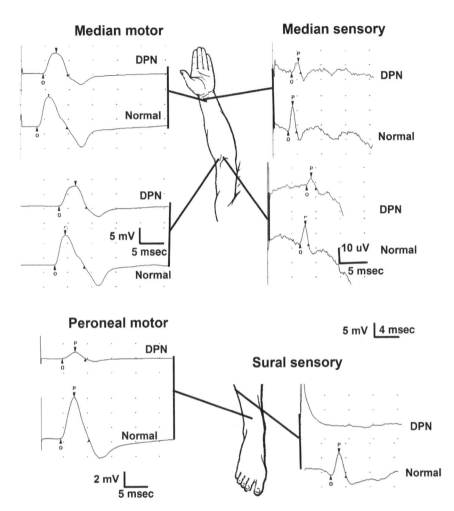

Figure 9.2 Nerve conduction abnormalities in a patient with moderately severe diabetic polyneuropathy compared to responses in a normal subject. Note that the motor responses (CMAPs) and sensory responses (SNAPs) in both the upper and lower limbs are reduced in amplitude and are delayed. The sural sensory potential is absent. Refer to the guide for normal studies in Figures 2.1 to 2.3.

- Possible causes include oxidative stress and nitrative stress (from oxygen- and nitrogen-based free radicals, respectively), abnormal signaling to neurons by advanced glycosylated end products (AGEs) through RAGE (receptor for AGEs), abnormal direct insulin signaling of neurons, loss of growth factors for neurons, excessive flux of polyols (sugar alcohols) through the aldose reductase pathway, chronic ischemia and hypoxia of nerve from microangiopathy (disease of small blood vessels supplying nerves and ganglia) (Table 9.2).

Table 9.2 Mechanisms Linked to the Development of Diabetic Polyneuropathy

Excessive flux through the polyol (sugar alcohol) pathway
Microangiopathy (disease of small blood vessels) involving peripheral nerves and ganglia
   with ischemia and hypoxia
Oxidative and nitrative stress from free radicals
Lack of trophic support of neurons from neurotrophic growth factors
Abnormal glycation of key neuronal proteins
Abnormal signaling by circulating advanced end products of glycosylation (AGEs)
   ligating AGE receptors (RAGE)
Abnormalities in direct insulin signaling of neurons
Combinations of the above mechanisms that target neurons while failing to offer
   appropriate support

TREATMENT

- Neuropathic pain therapy (see chap. 8).
- No treatments definitively arrest or reverse polyneuropathy.
- Daily foot inspection for injuries and early ulceration is mandatory.
- Several clinical trials suggest benefits from aldose reductase inhibitors (ARIs) but the data are inconclusive [see Cochrane review; (60)]; α-lipoic acid appeared beneficial in several trials but the overall results are not conclusive; C-peptide (portion of insulin promolecule) shows early benefits in clinical trials.
- Negative (no benefit) trials: PKCβ inhibitor (ruboxistaurin), growth factors (NGF, BDNF), acetyl-L-carnitine.
- Tight control of hyperglycemia reduces the incidence and progression of DPN in type 1 diabetes [DCCT trial (61)]; similar findings have also been confirmed in type 2 diabetes mellitus.
- Treat modifiable risk factors (obesity, smoking, hypertension).

10

Entrapment neuropathies

Damage to individual peripheral nerve trunks, known as focal neuropathies or mononeuropathies, are common in diabetic patients. Some of these neuropathies are thought to arise from direct compression, or entrapment, of nerves at specific sites in the limb that are vulnerable. Entrapment neuropathies are an important cause of disability in patients.

KEY POINTS

- Entrapment neuropathies are common in both type 1 and 2 diabetes mellitus.
- They may be mistaken for polyneuropathy and not specifically treated.
- They can be associated with significant neuropathic pain.
- They are a common cause of work-related disability.
- Nerve conduction studies are essential for diagnosis.
- Surgical decompression should be carefully considered and only carried out by experienced plastic surgeons, hand surgeons or neurosurgeons.

CARPAL TUNNEL SYNDROME

KEY POINTS

- Presents with tingling of fingers, especially at night or on awakening, driving.
- Patients flail or shake their hands to relieve symptoms.
- May be associated with painful tingling, wrist pain, or radiating arm pain.
- May or may not have objective loss to sensation on testing.
- Tinel's sign (tapping over median nerve to evoke paraesthesiae) is not always positive.
- Worse with pregnancy, manual or unaccustomed work, associated connective tissue disorders, hypothyroidism, acromegaly, female gender.
- May benefit from a wrist splint.

Clinical Features

Carpal tunnel syndrome (CTS) develops from entrapment of the median nerve at the wrist beneath the transverse carpal ligament. Repetitive use of the wrist (flexion and extension) predispose to its development. It is associated with positive sensory symptoms and pain in the territory of the median nerve (thumb, index, middle and lateral side of ring finger). Many patients complain of symptoms in all digits of their hand. Symptoms may be prominent at night or on awakening. Mild CTS may be associated with only symptoms whereas moderate or severe CTS may have clinical signs of sensory loss and thenar (especially lateral thenar) weakness. Concurrent hypothyroidism, pregnancy and rheumatoid arthritis are other predisposing conditions beyond diabetes. CTS may be combined with mild lower limb polyneuropathy erroneously suggesting more widespread polyneuropathy. Electrophysiological studies can clarify whether CTS is superimposed (see below). It is important that clinicians retain a high index of suspicion that treatable CTS may be identified in diabetic patients who also have polyneuropathy. CTS may also emerge later because of increased use of the hands in patients with polyneuropathy when walking is difficult. Longer standing and more severe CTS may be associated with hand weakness from thenar muscle denervation and wasting. Asymptomatic CTS (electrophysiological diagnosis) can be detected in 20% to 30% of diabetics but symptomatic CTS in present in approximately 6% of diabetics (57,68) (Table 10.1). It is the most common entrapment neuropathy overall and the most common type in diabetic subjects. Women are afflicted more than men and the dominant hand more than the nondominant.

Diagnosis

- Clinical findings of sensory loss in part of (e.g., distal digit tips), or all of the median nerve territory: thumb, index, middle, lateral ring finger, dorsal ends of the above fingers, lateral volar hand to the wrist (a small portion of the distal thenar eminence is spared since it is supplied by the palmar cutaneous branch that arises proximal to the carpal tunnel) (Fig. 10.1).
- Tinel's sign (tapping over the median nerve at the wrist evokes positive sensory symptoms that resemble the patient's symptoms and that are distal to the wrist, in the median territory) and Phalen's sign (both wrists flexed and held against each other for one minute) signs may be present. Both

Table 10.1   Dyck/Mayo Staging for the Severity of CTS

0: No clinical or electrophysiological evidence
1: Electrophysiological but not clinical evidence
2a: Clinical features with or without electrophysiological findings
2b: Clinical and diagnostic electrophysiological features of CTS

Abbreviation: CTS, carpal tunnel syndrome.
Source: From Ref. 57 with permission.

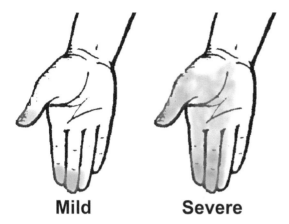

Mild   Severe

Figure 10.1 Illustration of progressive sensory changes in the hand of a patient with carpal tunnel syndrome. The changes may represent symptoms, such as pain or paraesthesiae (tingling) or loss of sensation. Note the sparing of the proximal part of the thenar eminence supplied by the palmar cutaneous branch of the median nerve that does not travel through the carpal tunnel.

tests can be unreliable however, having a significant number of false positives and false negatives.
- There may be weakness or thumb abduction by the abductor pollicus brevis (APB) and thenar wasting in severe CTS. In mild CTS, clinical signs may be absent.
- CTS is distinguished from C7 radiculopathy by the absence of neck pain radiating down the arm, the presence of an intact triceps reflex (supplied by C7 and lost in a C7 radiculopathy) and the absence of weakness of other C7 muscles. In a C6 radiculopathy with thumb numbness, there is loss of the biceps and brachioradialis reflex, C6 muscle weakness and radiating neck pain.
- Electrophysiological studies: several approaches are recommended to verify the diagnosis of CTS: (*i*) a *prolonged distal median nerve motor latency* across the carpal tunnel (stimulation at the wrist, recording over the APB); this should be compared with a normal distal latency from the ulnar nerve [stimulation at the wrist and recording over the abductor digiti minimi (ADM)]; (*ii*) *slowing of sensory conduction velocity* across the carpal tunnel with stimulation at the wrist and recording over the index, middle or ring fingers; this should be compared with normal sensory conduction from ulnar nerve stimulation and recording over the small (fifth) digit, or ring finger, and also compared with normal radial nerve sensory conduction stimulating at the distal forearm and recording over the radial sensory branch at the anatomical snuff box; (*iii*) *slowing of median palmar conduction* across the carpal tunnel (stimulation of the median nerve in the palm, recording over the median nerve at the wrist) compared

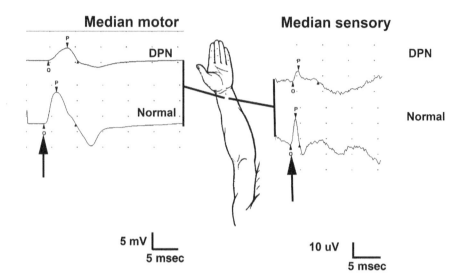

Figure 10.2 Nerve conduction abnormalities in a diabetic patient with CTS compared with responses in a normal subject. Note the delay in the motor response (CMAP), known as a prolonged distal motor latency. In this patient, the CMAP is also reduced in amplitude but this feature is not routinely identified in all instances of CTS. The sensory potentials (SNAPs) are also delayed and reduced in amplitude, features typical of CTS. For guidance with interpretation, refer to Figures 2.2 and 2.3. *Abbreviation*: CTS, carpal tunnel syndrome.

with normal ulnar conduction from the palm to the ulnar nerve at the wrist; and (*iv*) *denervation of median innervated hand muscles* (e.g., APB) with sparing of ulnar hand muscles (in more severe cases only).

- Electrophysiological studies to diagnose CTS should at least include: bilateral two point (wrist, elbow) median motor and sensory conduction, bilateral three point (wrist, below elbow, above elbow) ulnar motor and sensory conduction, bilateral radial sensory conduction, bilateral median and ulnar palmar conduction. Proximal stimulation for sensory nerves is not done in all laboratories (Fig. 10.2).

Treatment

- CTS may improve with a change in activity; spontaneous recovery may occur if it is secondary to short term overuse.
- Wrist splints worn at night and if possible during the day are beneficial; partial wrist immobilization with flexor bandaging may be used for day use if a splint is not practical.
- Decompression by section of the transverse carpal ligament by an experienced hand surgeon is the only curative procedure. Use of endoscopic release is controversial because of potential damage to the recurrent median motor branch. Steroid injections and use of pyridoxine are also

controversial. There is no evidence for benefit from various manipulation strategies (e.g., "active release" therapy).

- Recovery in diabetics, particularly those poorly controlled, may be less robust than in nondiabetics.
- CTS initially present during pregnancy may recur later with hand use.

ULNAR NEUROPATHY AT THE ELBOW

KEY POINTS

- Ulnar neuropathy at the elbow (UNE) can lead to progressive disability from hand weakness.
- Presents with numbness and tingling of the small fingers.
- May develop postoperatively.
- Elbow resting on chairs, vehicle doors or a bed are risk factors.
- A "Heelbo" pad, a padded arm sock fitted over the elbow, protects the nerve.
- The role for surgery is controversial.

Clinical Features

UNE can be debilitating when motor axons are involved because of its impact on hand function. Without motor involvement however, UNE may present with pain and positive or negative sensory symptoms in the small and medial half of the ring finger, radiating into the palm as far proximal as the wrist (only). There may be pain at the elbow. Asymptomatic slowing of ulnar motor conduction across the elbow is common in diabetic patients. Motor involvement causes wasting and weakness of intrinsic ulnar innervated hand muscles (ADM, interosseous muscles, ulnar lumbrical muscles, opponens pollicis), especially the first dorsal interosseous muscle. Manipulation of the ulnar nerve at the elbow may generate tingling that radiates into the hand, small and medial half of the ring finger. Patients with increased carrying angles of the arm (limitation of full elbow extension) are at greater risk for UNE as are patients that use excessive ethanol. The most common cause may be excessive leaning of the arm on the medial elbow, on a desk, chair or door of an automobile. The prevalence of UNE in patients with diabetes mellitus is estimated to be approximately 2% (68).

Diagnosis

- Clinical features of sensory loss in the ulnar nerve territory [small (fifth) finger, medial half of ring finger, medial volar and dorsal hand as far proximal as the wrist], and weakness of ulnar innervated muscles (ADM— weakness of small finger abduction; dorsal interossei—weakness of finger spread, and of adduction).

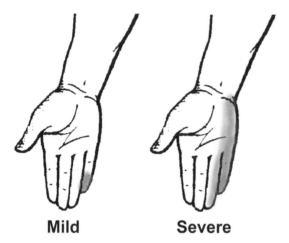

Mild   **Severe**

Figure 10.3 Illustration of progressive sensory changes in the hand of a patient with ulnar neuropathy at the elbow. The changes may represent symptoms such as pain or paraesthesiae (tingling) or loss of sensation. The medial forearm is not involved by ulnar neuropathy.

- Normal strength in C8-T1 muscles not innervated by the ulnar nerve such as APB and flexor pollicis longus.
- Sensory loss that also includes the medial forearm fully or part way up to the elbow does not occur in UNE but instead suggests a C8 radiculopathy.
- Electrophysiological studies: (*i*) *slowing of ulnar motor conduction* across the elbow; (*ii*) slowing of ulnar sensory conduction across the elbow, or loss of the ulnar SNAP across the elbow (proximal sensory studies are not performed in all laboratories); (*iii*) *conduction block or dispersion* of the ulnar CMAP across the elbow; (*iv*) *selective loss of the ulnar SNAP*; and (*v*) *denervation of ulnar innervated hand muscles* (e.g., first dorsal interosseous) with sparing of median innervated hand muscles; more proximal muscles such as flexor carpi ulnaris are also often spared in UNE (Fig. 10.3).

Treatment

- There are no controlled clinical trials in patients (diabetics or nondiabetics) that demonstrate decompression, compared with conservative management (change in positioning, Heelbo pad), improves long term outcome in diabetic patients.
- Current clinical practice suggests decompression; several types of surgery are available but none are known to be superior: ulnar transposition, medial epicondylectomy, in situ decompression without epicondylectomy, or decompression distal to the elbow by sectioning the flexor carpi ulnaris

aponeurosis just distal to the cubital tunnel (where entrapment beneath its edge can occur with elbow flexion); surgery is appropriate if there is progressive hand weakness that has not responded to conservative management.

- Electrophysiological studies may help guide whether release is appropriate: denervation of the ulnar innervated hand muscles that is not improving, frank conduction block at the elbow (indicating a local demyelinating lesion) that does not resolve with conservative therapy and progresses to axonal degeneration of the nerve.

PERONEAL NEUROPATHY AT KNEE

KEY POINTS

- Peroneal neuropathy at the knee presents with foot drop.
- Risk factors are leg crossing, prolonged squatting, and local injury or compression near the fibular head.
- Must be distinguished from L5 root compression in the lumbar spine.
- Role for surgical decompression is controversial.

Clinical Features

Common peroneal neuropathy at the fibular head is a common cause of foot drop. Patients are unable to dorsiflex the foot and toe fully or to evert the foot (turn it outward). There is sensory loss to light touch, temperature and pinprick over the dorsum of the foot. There is also sensory loss up the lateral aspect of the leg below the knee. Pain is less common. In longstanding cases, there may be wasting of the extensor digitorum brevis (EDB) muscle and in severe neuropathies, of the anterior compartment of the lower leg (tibialis anterior and extensor hallucis longus). At the fibular head, the most common site of compression, the peroneal nerve divides into deep and superficial branches. The deep peroneal branch supplies extensors of the foot and toes. It supplies sensation to the web space between the large and second toe. The superficial branch travels laterally to supply the muscles that evert the foot (peroneus longus and brevis) and its distal branch supplies the dorsum of the foot. Compression most commonly involves the common peroneal nerve with both dorsiflexion and eversion weakness. Activities that predispose to the development of peroneal neuropathy include injury to the lateral side of the knee, knee surgery, prolonged or habitual leg crossing, weight loss (thought to be due to loss of protective subcutaneous fat around the nerve), unrecognized compression during anesthesia and prolonged squatting (e.g., in roofers, or strawberry pickers—"strawberry picker's palsy"). Sometimes peroneal neuropathy may be a component of more widespread diabetic lumbosacral plexopathy (see chap. 12). Foot drop predisposes patients to falling because they catch their toes on carpets, curbs and other obstacles when they walk, causing them to pitch or fall forward. Some diabetic patients have been reported with bilateral peroneal entrapment neuropathies.

Diagnosis

- Clinical diagnosis is important: foot and toe dorsiflexion weakness, weakness of eversion but not of inversion, preservation of the ankle reflex (inversion weakness suggests L5 radiculopathy instead of peroneal neuropathy; ankle reflex involvement suggests the disorder is more widespread than the peroneal nerve alone—possible sciatic lesion), tingling and loss of sensation over the dorsum of the foot and lateral leg.
- There should be normal muscle strength in proximal L5 root territory muscles such as gluteus medius that abducts the hip.
- L5 radiculopathies have less severe foot, toe dorsiflexion and eversion weakness, but also have inversion weakness; there may be back pain and a positive straight leg raising sign (Lasègue's sign). Cauda equina lesions may compress multiple lumbar and sacral roots including fibers that supply bladder function.
- Loss of the ankle reflex and weakness of knee flexion with a foot drop suggest a more proximal sciatic lesion with prominent involvement of its peroneal fiber branches.
- Patients with cerebral infarction (or spinal cord disease) also have foot drop but it is accompanied by spasticity, brisk reflexes, an upgoing toe and often weakness in other lower limb muscles.
- MR imaging of the lumbar intraspinal space important to rule out L45 disk with L5 root compression or a laterally placed L5S1 disk with L5 root compression.
- Electrophysiological studies often show loss of the CMAP recorded over the EDB muscle compared with the contralateral side and loss of the superficial peroneal SNAP compared with the contralateral side (unless bilateral). Tibial motor conduction and sural sensory conduction in the involved limb should be normal. Peroneal motor conduction studies may identify conduction block, temporal dispersion and conduction slowing (any combination of the above) across the fibular head. In a relatively pure demyelinating peroneal neuropathy, the distal CMAP over EDB may be preserved with block, dispersion and slowing across the fibular head causing weakness of peroneal innervated muscles and sensory loss; Three point (ankle, below fibular head, and above fibular head) motor conduction studies are essential. Loss of the tibial CMAP and sural SNAP suggest a sciatic lesion. Needle EMG may show signs of denervation in the foot extensors (e.g., tibialis anterior) and toe extensors (e.g., EDB) as well as lateral peroneal muscles. Denervation of the gastrocnemius, tibialis posterior muscles, respectively, suggests a sciatic lesion or an L5

radiculopathy. Denervation of the short head of the biceps muscle as well as peroneal muscles indicate involvement of the peroneal fascicles of the sciatic nerve more proximally. Denervation of L5 paraspinal muscles indicates an L5 radiculopathy.

Treatment

- There is no evidence to support decompression of the peroneal nerve at the knee and it is uncommon to perform it in clinical practice.
- There is no role or evidence for multiple decompression procedures (including the peroneal nerve) that have been advocated for the treatment of diabetic polyneuropathy.
- Conservative therapy is recommended (avoid leg crossing, avoid compression of the side of the knee).
- Use of an ankle foot orthosis is important to reduce the risk of falling; fitting must be considerate of pressure points to prevent orthosis-related skin ulceration.

LATERAL FEMORAL CUTANEOUS NERVE OF THE THIGH (MERALGIA PARAESTHETICA)

KEY POINTS

- Meralgia paraesthetica presents with numbness and tingling of the lateral thigh.
- Risk factors are abdominal obesity, recent weight gain, tight low riding belts, pregnancy.
- The knee reflex on the same side is preserved, and there is no motor weakness.
- Must be distinguished from lumbosacral plexopathy, L3 or L4 root compression (radiculopathy).
- There is no evidence to support a role for surgical decompression.

Clinical Features

Meralgia paraesthetica arises from entrapment of the lateral femoral cutaneous nerve of the thigh under the inguinal ligament. Patients experience numbness, tingling, prickling and sometimes pain over the lateral thigh. Pain is often more widespread than the actual sensory deficit and may radiate up the leg and below the knee. The symptoms are related to leg posture or walking and may be relieved by sitting which reduces the stretch or tension on the nerve. There may be prominent allodynia with discomfort from garments over the thigh. Sensory testing identifies loss to light touch and pinprick over the lateral thigh. The exact territory may vary from a small patch over the lateral thigh to most of the lateral thigh from just below the inguinal area to the knee. Sensory loss should generally not be identified below the knee. Since this nerve supplies only sensation to the skin, motor power is preserved in hip flexion and knee extension. The knee reflex (quadriceps reflex) should also be preserved and comparable to that of the opposite side. In some instances however, meralgia paraesthetica may accompany severe diabetic polyneuropathy with diffuse loss of deep tendon reflexes. Some patients may have a Tinel's sign over the inguinal ligament such that tapping over the nerve, as it passes through the ligament, generates tingling in its cutaneous distribution. Palpation over the nerve at this level may also identify a compressive lesion such as an enlarged lymph node, an inguinal hernia or a scar from a previous hernia repair. Additional risk factors are abdominal obesity, pregnancy and the wearing of low riding belts. Meralgia paraesthetica from diabetes may be bilateral.

Diagnosis

- The diagnosis is primarily clinical with sensory loss in the lateral thigh, preserved thigh muscle function, and either a normal knee reflex or one comparable to the opposite side.
- The differential diagnosis includes diabetic lumbosacral plexopathy (usually motor, includes wasting, loss of reflexes), plexopathy secondary to retroperitoneal lesion (retroperitoneal tumor, psoas hematoma, or abscess) or an L3 or L4 radiculopathy (back pain, weakness, straight leg raising sign, loss of knee reflex).
- Imaging studies (MR of lumbosacral intraspinal space and pelvis, CT of pelvis) to exclude lumbar disk or a retroperitoneal lesion should be normal. They are only indicated if the clinical features are atypical.
- Electrophysiological studies are useful to exclude radiculopathy, plexopathy because these lesions may have denervation of L3, L4 innervated muscles; in meralgia paraesthetica, the CMAP of the vastus medialis should be normal and symmetric; SNAPs recorded from the lateral cutaneous nerve of the thigh may be lost in meralgia paraesthetica, but these are technically difficult to record and less reliable (Fig. 10.4).

Treatment

- There is no evidence to support surgical decompression at the thigh.
- In clinical practice patients may choose to undergo decompression if weight loss or local anesthetic or steroid injections are unhelpful and pain is intractable (69).
- Conservative management, including treatment of pain and limiting activities that provoke symptoms may be associated with spontaneous recovery over time.

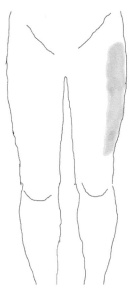

Figure 10.4 Illustration of the distribution of pain, paraesthesiae, or sensory loss in a patient with an entrapment of the lateral cutaneous nerve of the thigh (meralgia paraesthetica).

LESS COMMON FOCAL ENTRAPMENT NEUROPATHIES

KEY POINTS

- The relationship between their development and diabetes mellitus is unclear.
- These neuropathes require neurological evaluation and electrophysiological studies to clarify localization, differential diagnosis.

Sciatic Neuropathy

- There are rare case reports concurrent with diabetes.
- Patients may present with foot drop but also have evidence of tibial, sural nerve involvement with loss of ankle reflex, plantar flexion weakness, knee flexion weakness.
- Risk factors: hip surgery, pelvic fractures, misplaced gluteal injections, possibly compression.

Radial Neuropathy

- There are rare case reports concurrent with diabetes.
- Patients may present with wrist and finger drop; with wrist drop, intrinsic hand weakness may seem more widespread than in the radial distribution. It is essential that the other innervated muscles by the median and ulnar

nerve are examined with the wrist flattened on a surface; patients with wrist extensor weakness from cerebral lesions have mild extensor weakness with hand clumsiness but usually also have weakness of other arm muscles, pronator drift, deep tendon reflexes that are brisker than the other side.

- Patients with radial neuropathy may have sensory loss and tingling in the dorsolateral aspect of the hand.
- Risk factors: humeral fractures at the spiral groove, blunt trauma and external compression.

Obturator Neuropathy

- There are rare case reports concurrent with diabetes.
- Patients present with hip adductor weakness.
- The obturator nerve may be involved in more widespread diabetic lumbosacral plexopathy (see chap. 12).
- Risk factors: pelvic trauma, pelvic lesions, obturator hernia, obstetrical trauma.

Other Entrapment Neuropathies

- A number of additional rare examples are described, but are of uncertain relationship to diabetes.
- See reference for a complete review of focal neuropathies:(70).

11

Focal neuropathies without entrapment

Several additional focal neuropathies, not clearly linked to a site of compression or entrapment, are described in this chapter. Some, for example, oculomotor palsy, may arise from ischemia, especially in the vulnerable center of the nerve trunk. Others, like intercostal and abdominal neuropathies, are of uncertain cause.

KEY POINTS

- Focal neuropathies or mononeuropathies may occur at sites that are not prone to compression; ischemia may be responsible for some of these lesions.
- Intense neuropathic pain from segmental thoracic intercostal or abdominal radicular neuropathies may be mistaken for an intrathoracic or abdominal emergency.
- Oculomotor (third cranial) neuropathy secondary to diabetes (pupillary sparing) should be distinguished from compression or bleeding due to an intracranial berry aneurysm.
- May develop despite only mild hyperglycemia.

THORACIC INTERCOSTAL AND ABDOMINAL RADICULAR (TRUNCAL) NEUROPATHY

KEY POINTS

- Presents with intense pain that radiates around the trunk, is usually superficial, and may resemble herpes zoster without a rash.
- Patients may or may not have an associated clinical sensory deficit.
- The pain has neuropathic qualities including burning and tingling.
- May involve several contiguous segments.

Clinical Features

Thoracic intercostal and abdominal radicular neuropathies can present with severe thoracic or abdominal wall pain that sometimes resembles a visceral emergency. The differential diagnosis is not extensive, but these neuropathies should be distinguished from herpes zoster without rash or less commonly, radiculopathy from a segmental structural lesion. In a structural (mass) lesion, pain and tingling may intensify by moving the spine or by coughing, sneezing or straining. There may also be signs of myelopathy in a structural lesion including weakness, spasticity, bowel and bladder difficulties, brisk lower limb reflexes, and upgoing plantar responses.

The intercostal and radicular neuropathies may span several contiguous segmental territories and may be bilateral (Fig. 11.1) (71). Sensory loss to light touch or pinprick may or may not be present. Sensory loss, especially if it involves several adjacent dermatomes, is more likely to occur in diabetic radicular neuropathy than herpes zoster without rash. Descriptors of the pain indicate a neuropathic etiology: tingling, pricking, lancinating, aching at night, radiation around the chest or abdomen causing a constricting feeling, and sometimes allodynia. Weight loss may occur, especially if the neuropathy accompanies lumbosacral plexopathy (see chap. 12). Patients may occasionally have asymptomatic sensory loss over the chest or abdomen from longer standing truncal or radicular neuropathy. There may be asymmetric weakness of abdominal muscles, detected by asking the patient to do a sit-up (asymmetric bulging). Males are involved more often. Radicular neuropathies may develop in either type 1 or 2 diabetes, and may be a presenting symptom of diabetes in older type 2 diabetic patients. The cause of diabetic truncal radiculopathies is unknown.

Diagnosis

- The diagnosis is usually based on clinical symptoms and signs; imaging of the spinal cord and roots with MR and gadolinium is indicated if there are atypical features or if a structural lesion is suspected.
- Electrophysiological studies may detect signs of generalized peripheral neuropathy.
- EMG may detect denervation (fibrillations, positive sharp waves) in weak thoracic intercostals or abdominal muscles. Care is required to avoid peritoneal or pleural penetration (pneumothorax) if the abdominal wall muscles or intercostal muscles are examined by needle EMG.

Treatment

- Deficits may slowly resolve over time.
- Pain management is usually required.
- It is uncertain whether glycemic control influences the development or resolution of diabetic radiculopathy.

Thoracic intercostal neuropathy

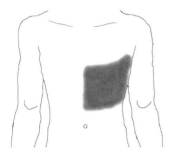

Abdominal neuropathy

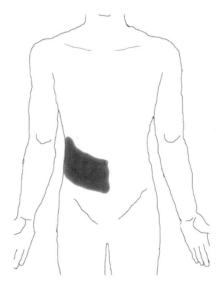

Figure 11.1 Illustration of the territory of pain, paraesthesiae, or sensory loss in patients with truncal neuropathy involving thoracic intercostal nerves (*above*) or abdominal cutaneous nerves (*below*). Truncal neuropathies often involve more than one contiguous nerve territory.

OCULOMOTOR PALSY (THIRD CRANIAL NERVE)

KEY POINTS

- Oculomotor palsy in diabetes usually spares the pupillary fibers, distinguishing it from pupillary involvement observed in compression from structural or mass lesions such as berry aneurysms or tumors.
- Sudden onset; may be painful.
- Hypertension is an additional risk factor.

Clinical Features

Oculomotor (third cranial nerve) neuropathy presents in patients with sudden diploplia and ptosis (eyelid drooping). An aching pain around or behind the eye often precedes the neurological deficit. Both ptosis and extraocular involvement are often incomplete. The eye is deviated laterally (abducted) because muscles of adduction are partly or fully paralyzed by the neuropathy. Up and down gaze in the involved eye are weak. Internal rotation and down gaze during attempted eye adduction may be spared, since both are movements that involve the superior oblique muscle innervated by the trochlear (fourth cranial) nerve. Diabetic oculomotor palsy may routinely spare the pupil because axons within the center of the nerve are the most vulnerable and are targeted, a feature of ischemic nerve damage. Pupillary fibers, normally responsible for pupil constriction, are found on the outer rim of the nerve and spared by ischemia. This concept is supported by a single pathological study (72) that noted demyelination in the center of the oculomotor nerve within the cavernous sinus. Other cranial nerves (see below) such as the sixth (abducens) or fourth (trochlear) cranial nerve may also be involved.

Diagnosis

- The clinical diagnosis is made from sudden onset of diploplia with eyelid drooping, weakness of eye adduction, elevation and depression; the pupil is usually intact.
- Imaging should include MR assessment of the brainstem and the course of the oculomotor nerve; MR angiography is indicated to search for evidence of an aneurysm compressing the third cranial nerve. CT angiography is also useful in diabetic patients but there is a risk of contrast nephropathy from the higher contrast loads used in this procedure (see chap. 4).
- Conventional carotid and vertebral angiography remain the gold standard to detect or exclude berry intracranial aneurysms; the procedure is invasive and requires iodinated contrast administration.
- If there are typical clinical features of diabetic oculomotor palsy (sudden onset, pain, pupillary sparing), noninvasive imaging (without a formal angiogram) may be sufficient to exclude a structural lesion or aneurysm.
- Myasthenia gravis may present with ptosis and extraocular palsy that spares the pupil; deficits are usually more variable and worse with fatigue or later in the day.

Treatment

- No specific treatment is available.
- Usually resolves spontaneously over approximately three months.
- An eye patch prevents diploplia but interrupts binocular depth vision.
- Patients should refrain from driving because of diploplia or loss of binocular depth vision if an eye patch is used.

FACIAL NEUROPATHY (SEVENTH CRANIAL NERVE)

KEY POINTS

- Facial neuropathy (Bell's palsy) is more common in diabetic patients.
- The facial palsy from neuropathy is important to distinguish from a CNS lesion that spares forehead movement (furrowing).
- Facial neuropathy may be associated with herpes zoster; zoster is associated with herpetic vesicles in the external canal, or palate on the side of the nerve lesion.

Clinical Features

The most common cause of facial neuropathy in the general population is Bell's palsy, a self-limited inflammatory disorder of the facial (seventh) cranial nerve. A subacute onset over several hours or on awakening is typical; it presents with asymmetry of facial movement that involves all parts of the face: forehead, eye closure, mouth, platysma in the neck. Eye closure weakness may be partial or complete. There may be associated facial pain and tingling sensations although sensory loss is generally not detected. Weakness of inner ear muscles supplied by the facial nerve may result in hyperacusis. Other symptoms include loss of taste in the anterior two-thirds of the tongue, and ipsilateral loss of lacrimation. Some cases of severe facial neuropathy associated with herpes zoster infection (Ramsay-Hunt syndrome) have herpes vesicles in the external canal or palate. Facial neuropathy is distinguished from cerebral or brainstem infarction by the involvement of the forehead muscles (spared in cerebral lesions) and absence of other deficits. Recovery usually occurs over weeks to months. Occasional patients may have severe deficits that do not recover. Patients with severe lesions and partial recovery may have aberrant reinnervation: motor fibers destined for some facial muscles inappropriately reinnervate alternate muscles. Aberrant reinnervation results in synkinesis, the inappropriate activation of incorrect facial muscles during facial movement, for example, blinking evokes mouth movements, mouth movements cause movements of the muscles around the eye (orbicularis oculus). An abnormal gustatolacrimal reflex may develop causing the patient to shed tears while eating, a phenomenon also known as "crocodile tears." Patients with severe facial nerve lesions and only limited recovery, may also develop contracture around their eye (contracture of the orbicularis oculus) with narrowing of their palpebral fissure.

Diagnosis

- The clinical diagnosis is identified by the development of subacute facial weakness with difficulty closing the eye, moving the mouth and wrinkling the forehead without sensory loss or weakness of other cranial nerves or limb muscles.

- Patients may also report pain over the mastoid process and loss or altered taste sensation.
- Testing of taste and finding unilateral loss of sweet sensation on the anterior two-thirds of the tongue helps to secure the diagnosis.
- Facial weakness with sparing of forehead wrinkling suggests a cerebral lesion.
- Noninvasive imaging (brain CT or MR) in typical cases is indicated to exclude other causes of facial paralysis including compressive tumors, vascular lesions or others.
- The presence of other cranial neuropathies is a "red flag" and requires careful imaging with contrast (e.g., brain MR with gadolinium) to exclude a base of skull structural lesion, base of skull inflammatory meningitis (TB, carcinomatous, or lymphomatous), or other causes of inflammation such as sarcoidosis.
- Electrophysiological studies are not required in all cases but may be helpful for more severe lesions; if postponed until at least 21 days after the onset, the studies can identify facial nerve axon loss with denervation. Severe axon loss has a less favorable prognosis for recovery. Facial nerve motor conduction studies may identify a low amplitude nasalis or orbicularis oculus CMAP (compared with the intact contralateral side) if there is axon loss and needle EMG may identify denervation with fibrillations and positive sharp waves in one or more facial muscles. EMG may also identify synkinesis. In early cases, blink reflex studies may be helpful. On stimulating the supraorbital sensory nerve on the side of the paralysis, the ipsilateral monosynaptic R1 response and R2 response may be delayed or absent whereas the contralateral polysynaptic R2 response is normal. On stimulating the nerve on the intact side, both R1 and R2 should be preserved ipsilaterally but the contralateral R2 response is delayed or absent.

Treatment

- In Bell's palsy, 75% of cases will recover in the first six weeks and 90% by three months. About 10% of patients will be left with residual facial nerve dysfunction characterized by weakness and later synkinesis, crocodile tears or contracture.
- A short course of prednisone (e.g., 60 mg for two days then tapering quickly over 10–14 days) may speed recovery but the benefit is modest. Therapy may only be warranted if it can be instituted quickly (within 48 hours of onset) and if the facial nerve palsy is complete. Facial paresis will recover spontaneously.
- There is no clear evidence that antiviral therapy improves outcome in nonzoster Bell's palsy; it may be for used in herpes zoster–related facial neuropathy (Ramsay-Hunt syndrome). Some consultants suggest that if the

risks of renal adverse events from the drug are low treatment can be started within 48 hours of onset, with a one week course of famciclovir or valacyclovir.

- Eye protection is indicated to prevent corneal ulceration due to drying, for example, tape eyelids shut, use artificial tears.
- Reference (73).

OTHER CRANIAL NEUROPATHIES

Abducens Palsy (Sixth Cranial Nerve)

- Abducens palsy may be as or more common than oculomotor palsy in older diabetic patients; other causes include compression, trauma and hypertension.
- Presents with eye pain, horizontal diploplia, weakness of abduction of one eye; spontaneous recovery normally occurs within three months.
- Noninvasive imaging (brain CT) is appropriate for excluding other causes in otherwise typical cases; suggestions are as above for oculomotor palsy for atypical cases or cases with other neurological symptoms (including more detailed cranial imaging as appropriate).
- The abducens nerve is highly susceptible to compression from a variety of intracranial lesions, and sixth nerve palsy is typically described as a "false localizing sign;" caution is advised including a thorough evaluation.

Trochlear Palsy (Fourth Cranial Nerve)

- Trochlear palsy presents with diploplia from difficulty looking down and inward because of weakness of superior oblique muscle.
- Patient tilts head to the side opposite to the palsy to reduce diploplia.
- Often associated with oculomotor palsy with inability to internally rotate the eye.
- Investigation, outcome as for oculomotor and abducens lesions.

12

Lumbosacral plexopathy

Diabetic lumbosacral plexopathy (DLSP) is an uncommon but debilitating complication, especially in older patients with type 2 diabetes. Previously described as "femoral neuropathy," it is a painful, subacute, largely motor disorder.

KEY POINTS

- Lumbosacral plexopathy is important to consider in diabetic patients with unexplained thigh pain.
- May develop in patients with only mild hyperglycemia; sometimes follows initiation of insulin therapy.
- Despite severe disability, partial or full recovery can occur in most patients.
- May involve the contralateral leg after several months.
- Often associated with severe weight loss (cachexia).
- Atypical forms (more distal weakness, bilateral involvement) can occur.
- Imaging of the lumbar intraspinal space and lumbosacral plexus is important to exclude an alternate cause (e.g., retroperitoneal tumor); MR is preferred and may detect signal change or atrophy in the denervated muscle.

Clinical Features

DLSP is also known as radiculoplexus neuropathy, diabetic amyotrophy, Bruns-Garland syndrome, and proximal diabetic neuropathy (74,75). This condition also overlaps with what is termed multifocal diabetic neuropathy: the difference is that upper limb and truncal involvement also occur in the latter condition. DLSP is typically diagnosed in patients with type 2 diabetes mellitus, more often in males and older diabetic subjects. DLSP may be a presenting feature of type 2 diabetes. It is a severe and disabling complication of diabetes associated with impairment in standing and walking and severe neuropathic pain. DLSP usually presents as a unilateral intense deep boring or aching muscle pain, sometimes worse at night, within the muscles of the thigh but also radiating to the back and perineum. In some patients, the pain may be superficial with paraesthesiae and burning. Pain usually precedes weakness and wasting of proximal thigh muscles over the next few weeks. The afflicted muscles include the quadriceps, ileopsoas, hip adductor muscles and occasionally, the anterior tibial muscles (with foot drop). Sensory loss or tingling can occur but they are often less prominent or absent. DLSP was once called femoral neuropathy because the muscles inner-vated by the femoral nerve are most often involved. DLSP also involves other thigh muscles such as the medial adductor muscles innervated by the obturator nerve, and the ileopsoas muscle innervated directly by the lumbar plexus. Many patients are unable to walk and require a wheelchair. Over months, slow recovery of muscle power occurs. In some patients, contralateral DLSP may emerge a few weeks later. Variations of DLSP include symmetrical involvement, foot drop or apparent worsening of generalized features of polyneuropathy. Surprisingly, it may emerge early in the course of diabetes or following institution of insulin therapy in type 2 diabetic patients. Nondiabetics can rarely develop a similar syndrome (76).

Pathological studies are few but one autopsy study identified occlusive changes in microvessels supplying the lumbosacral plexus (77). More recent studies have identified perivascular inflammation, epineurial inflammation, microvessel occlusion and iron deposition, indicative of intraneural bleeding, in biopsies of the sural nerve or thigh cutaneous nerves (intermediate cutaneous nerve of the thigh); all of these features are suggestive of a form of vasculitis, an autoimmune inflammation of blood vessels (78,79). Despite these inflammatory changes, the response to immunosuppressive therapy is not clear or robust. Nerve biopsies also identify loss of myelinated and unmyelinated axons.

Diagnosis

- The clinical diagnosis is made by the history of a subacute severe unilateral deep boring thigh pain, followed over days to weeks by thigh muscle weakness and atrophy with loss of the ipsilateral knee reflex and lesser sensory involvement.
- Imaging studies of the lumbar intraspinal space (MR with gadolinium) and the lumbosacral plexus [MR with gadolinium or CT with contrast (see concerns about contrast complications, chap. 3)] are indicated to help to exclude a compressive plexus lesion such as a retroperitoneal tumor or hematoma.
- Patients with L3, L4 radiculopathies are expected to have more prominent back pain radiating into the thigh, with more prominent sensory symptoms and findings.
- Electrophysiological studies may identify loss of the amplitude of the CMAP recorded over a quadriceps muscle (e.g., vastus medialis) compared

with that of the uninvolved contralateral side; denervation (fibrillations, positive sharp waves) may be detected in quadriceps, ileopsoas, hip adductors, lumbar and sacral paraspinal muscles and occasionally in more widespread muscles, for example, tibialis anterior. Nerve conduction studies may identify evidence of widespread polyneuropathy. Enlarged motor units, indicating early collateral reinnervation, may be detected during recovery of the proximal leg muscles.

Treatment

- No therapy is yet available to arrest or reverse the motor deficit.
- Preliminary data suggests that an intravenous course of glucocorticoid may shorten the duration of pain associated with DLSP but not its disability (Dyck et al., unpublished data).
- There is no evidence of benefit from IVIG.
- Patients require intensive pain management and therapy may include opioids.
- Patients require physiotherapy and occupational therapy during recovery; a knee brace to prevent buckling when weight bearing may be helpful.

13

Diabetic autonomic neuropathy

Diabetic autonomic neuropathy (DAN) is common but often undetected. A thorough laboratory-based workup of DAN is often not available, although some forms of evaluation may be carried out in EMG laboratories. Erectile dysfunction (ED) in males may be the most common symptom of DAN.

KEY POINTS

- Diabetic autonomic neuropathy (DAN) is associated with an increased risk of cardiovascular mortality.
- The most common symptom of DAN is erectile dysfunction in men.
- DAN may present with minimal DPN.
- Primary autonomic targets are sweating, cardiovascular, sexual function, upper and lower gastrointestinal (GI) motility.
- All diabetic patients should be questioned about autonomic symptoms.
- Routinely check blood pressure (BP) and pulse supine, then standing at one minute for postural hypotension (abnormal systolic drop of 20 mmHg or greater).
- Medications can exacerbate postural hypotension and bladder urinary retention.
- DAN is associated with "silent" cardiac abnormalities including abnormal cardiac contractility, "silent ischemia," or myocardial infarction.

CLINICAL FEATURES

Cardiovascular Abnormalities

- Patients may have a fixed mildly elevated heart rate that is asymptomatic (e.g., 90–100 bpm) and that resembles a transplanted heart (that lacks a nerve supply).

- Abnormal innervation of the heart may theoretically contribute to abnormal contractility and arrhythmias.
- Postural hypotension is defined as a drop of systolic pressure of 20 mmHg or more after one minute of standing, with orthostatic dizziness or fainting; it results from loss of sympathetic control to resistance arterioles. Postural hypotension occurs in 3% to 6% of diabetics (80) and may be a later feature of DAN. Some patients may have abnormal tachycardia with standing (POTS, postural orthostatic tachycardia syndrome).
- Although largely asymptomatic, diabetic patients have loss of RR (heart rate) interval variability at rest, with Valsalva, standing, and other maneuvers.
- Prolonged QT_c (corrected QT) intervals in type I diabetics may predict an increased risk of mortality (81).
- There may be a higher prevalence of obstructive sleep apnea in diabetic patients.

Sexual Dysfunction

- Male ED may occur in over 40% of diabetic men (82). It is defined as the inability to achieve or maintain an erection sufficient for sexual intercourse (83). ED is a common manifestation of autonomic neuropathy in males. Direct vascular factors, such as atherosclerosis, also cause ED. Other causes should be excluded: psychogenic ED, Peyronie's disease, problems of the sexual partner, and medications (sedatives, antidepressants, antihypertensives). The additional loss of ejaculation suggests more severe autonomic involvement.
- Female sexual dysfunction may occur from vaginitis, loss of vaginal lubrication, cystitis, and other causes.

Gastrointestinal Problems

- Overall symptoms that are more common in diabetic patients include abdominal pain, weight loss, postprandial fullness, heartburn, nausea (rarely vomiting), dysphagia, fecal incontinence, diarrhea, and constipation (38).
- Esophageal transit is slowed and lower sphincter pressure reduced. Patients may have dysphagia with heartburn and rarely esophageal ulceration and stricture formation.
- Gastric emptying is slowed. There is a direct relationship between glucose levels and gastric emptying; an improvement of glucose levels in poorly controlled diabetics may increase emptying. A direct relationship also exists between postprandial declines in blood pressure and gastric emptying. Early satiety, pain, nausea, and delayed absorption of medications are results of delayed gastric emptying. There is a long list of disorders that also cause delayed gastric emptying (e.g., medications, electrolyte abnormalities, hypothyroidism, myotonic dystrophy, amyloidosis, postsurgical, and others).

- Small-intestine dysmotility may be associated with diarrhea. There is an increased risk of cholelithiasis and cholecystitis in diabetes from altered motility, abnormal sphincter of Oddi function, and abnormal bile composition.
- Colonic dysfunction causes constipation, diarrhea, and abdominal pain. Constipation and constipation alternating with diarrhea, sometimes nocturnal, can occur.
- Anorectal dysfunction with incontinence develops from abnormal internal or external sphincter function, loss of sensitivity, and disrupted anorectal reflexes. As in gastric emptying, sphincter dysfunction may be directly related to hyperglycemia. A superimposed history of obstetrical trauma may predispose diabetic women to this complication.
- Exclusion of other GI problems is important, including esophageal candidiasis, gastric bezoar, *Helicobacter pylori* infection, bacterial overgrowth, anorectal disorders, and celiac disease. Rectal examination is essential to exclude local abnormalities that may confound the diagnosis such as hemorrhoids, impaired sphincter tone, rectal prolapse, local tumors, local ulcers, rectal intussusception, and fecal impaction.

Bladder Dysfunction

- Loss of bladder sensitivity leads to overflow incontinence. Both sensory neuropathy and later efferent fiber dysfunction (detrusor muscle weakness) contribute to the "diabetic bladder." There is incomplete bladder emptying, recurrent infection, eventual overflow incontinence, and an end-stage insensitive noncontractile atonic bladder.
- Bladder irritability with urgency, nocturia, and incontinence can occur in some patients.
- Other urological problems such as bladder tumor, urethral stricture, prostatic hypertrophy, or tumor should be excluded. A rectal examination to detect prostatic hypertrophy or tumor is important.

Abnormalities of Sweating (Sudomotor Neuropathy)

- Symptoms of sudomotor DAN include loss of sweating (anhidrosis) in the feet, then hands in a stocking and glove distribution. Dry feet increase the risk of skin ulceration, and generalized loss of sweating may increase heat intolerance.
- Abnormal patterns of sweating in other areas of the body may occur, as documented by the thermoregulatory sweat testing (TST) test (see later in text). This includes inappropriate truncal sweating, other types of increased sweating (hyperhidrosis), or gustatory sweating.
- Gustatory sweating refers to facial and trunk sweating precipitated by eating certain foods such as hot or spicy dishes (84).

Other Symptoms

- *Pupils:* Diabetic persons may have small pupils from autonomic dysfunction. Pupillary reflexes may be sluggish or occasionally absent. There may be light intolerance from impaired pupillary reflexes. Ophthalmological assessment is required to identify diabetic retinopathy and other disorders.
- *Hypoglycemic unawareness:* Patients may have unawareness of their hypoglycemia because autonomic responses (sweating, tachycardia) and counterregulatory hormones such as epinephrine fail to rise. Since cognitive dysfunction can occur at glucose levels less than 2.7 mmol/L (50 mg/dL) and counteracting glucagon levels may fail to rise, patients may not recognize their impairment or to take adequate protective measures.
- *Loss of exercise capacity* may in part be related to autonomic neuropathy.

DIAGNOSTIC METHODS

- Supine and standing (one minute) BP (normal <20 mmHg systolic drop) and pulse (or formal tilt table testing).
- Changes in heart rate (RR interval) variability: resting heart rate, deep breathing, Valsalva, standing, mental arithmetic, inspiratory gasp (*these can be done using most modern EMG equipment*); see Ref. 85 for reference values.
- The Ewing battery (86,87) is a traditional set of cardiovascular autonomic tests: (*i*) Heart rate response to the Valsalva maneuver (normal maximum/minimum RR interval > 1.21); (*ii*) heart rate response to standing up (30:15 ratio—ratio of RR interval at 30th beat vs. 15 beat after standing; normal >1.04); (*iii*) heart rate response to deep breathing (normal variation >15 bpm); (*iv*) BP response to standing up (normal systolic fall <10 mmHg; abnormal is >20 mmHg); (*v*) BP response to sustained handgrip (normal should rise >16 mmHg systolic BP).
- These studies can be influenced by age, concurrent cardiovascular disease, and medications. Careful standardization of testing conditions is required. A recent consensus conference indicated that RR changes to deep breathing, RR change during Valsalva maneuver, and measurement of postural BP are the three most validated tests of cardiac autonomic dysfunction (88).
- Other less widely used autonomic tests of cardiovascular function: RR and BP changes to sustained handgrip, cold pressor (hand in ice water), squatting or rising from squatting, baroreflex sensitivity, QT_c (corrected QT) interval or dispersion, 24-hour RR interval variability (heart rate variability; including frequency analysis), and radionuclide imaging of cardiac contractility.
- Increases in the QT_c interval or its dispersion may be predictors of cardiac death. Impaired baroreflex sensitivity correlates with abnormal heart rate variability and postural hypotension.
- Radioiodinated metaiodobenzylguanidine (MIBG) is an injectable marker of sympathetic terminals found in cardiac muscle; loss of MIBG uptake in the inferior, posterior, and apical portions of the heart occurs in diabetes, indicating sympathetic denervation or dysfunction.

- Gastric and intestinal motility studies: assessment of esophageal function by transit studies using radiography or scintigraphy, by lower sphincter manometry, esophageal pH recordings and by endoscopy. Gastric function can be assessed by emptying studies using scintigraphy (dual isotopes can measure liquid and solid emptying) and endoscopy. Small intestinal dysfunction is studied by manometry, H_2-lactulose breath test, and gall bladder stones detected by ultrasound (including dynamic ultrasonography). Colon function is assessed by transit investigations using radiopaque studies or scintigraphy and by colonoscopy. Anorectal dysfunction is studied by manometry, ultrasonography, colonic transit, radiography, proctoscopy, and sigmoidoscopy.
- For ED evaluation: duplex ultrasonography, response to intracavernous injection, nocturnal measurements of penile tumescence (distinguishes psychogenic ED that has normal nocturnal tumescence).
- For bladder dysfunction: a urodynamic workup with cystometrogram, urinary tract imaging (e.g., intravenous pyelography), cystography and uroflowmetry, and postvoid ultrasonography to test for residual urine.
- For analysis of sweating: (*i*) thermoregulatory sweat testing (TST) examines the geographical distribution of sweating on the body; TST involves placing the patient in a heat cradle, raising the body temperature by 1.0°C, and painting the body with a sweat indicator (originally starch and iodine that turns black on sweating; more recently with alizarin red (89)); (*ii*) QSART (quantitative sudomotor axon reflex testing; less widely available) tests quantitative sweat output using a dehumidified sweat capsule; the setup delivers acetylcholine by iontophoresis (an electrical method to allow the molecule to penetrate the skin) to stimulate local sweat secretion on an upper and lower limb. In diabetes, QSART output may be reduced, absent, excessive, or "hung up" (persistent); (*iii*) SSR (sympathetic skin response) is a slow onset, broad peak electrical discharge that can be recorded in the hand in response to contralateral electrical stimulation, or a sudden inspiratory gasp; it is thought to arise from the synchronous activation of sweat glands; (*iv*) other measures of sweat output: analysis of sweat droplet numbers (numbers of functioning sweat glands) and size (90), skin biopsy to analyze sweat gland innervation (91), and novel rapid sweat indicator commercial methods (92). Overall, quantitative tests of sweat output and distribution are only available in some centers.
- Pupils may be analyzed by pupillograms (infared, darkness videopupillometry to measure pupillary diameter, latency to contraction, contraction, and dilation velocity).

TREATMENT

- Discontinue or reduce doses of medications that cause postural hypotension (e.g., tricyclic antidepressants, antihypertensive medications, other vasodilators).

- Implement BP checks for postural hypotension (calibrated with a mercury, or office standard); check and record supine then upright several times per day and record the result.
- Arise from bed or chair slowly; use a walker chair to sit down if dizziness develops outside of the home; sleep with the head of bed raised 20°; avoid prolonged standing, early morning or postprandial exercise; avoid prolonged heat exposure, hot baths, Jacuzzis, or hot showers.
- Increase salt and fluid intake; limit alcohol intake.
- Medications for postural hypotension: Fluorinef (dose range 0.1–0.4 mg) to increase fluid retention (watch for supine hypertension); midodrine (dose range 2.5–10 mg three times daily)—take doses while upright to avoid postural hypertension and omit doses before bedtime; DDAVP (dose range 5–40 µg intranasal at bedtime)—monitor for hyponatremia; investigational-L-threo-DOPS, octreotide.
- Screen for other causes of ED, including depression, medications, prostate disease, others.
- For esophageal dysphagia, consume liquids after solid meals to reduce the risk of ulceration. The therapeutic benefits of prokinetic drugs are uncertain.
- High-fiber, low-fat diet may facilitate gastric emptying.
- Pharmacological treatments of slowed gastric emptying include prokinetic agents [domperidone, metoclopramide, erythromycin (including intravenous dosing)]. Cisapride has been withdrawn from the market in many countries because of cardiac arrhythmia and death.
- For intractable impaired gastric emptying, a temporary or permanent jejunostomy may rarely be required.
- For intestinal motility problems (diarrhea), consider opiods (loperamide, codeine), cholestryramine, fiber, and bulking agents.
- Biofeedback may help with fecal incontinence.
- For male ED, consider phosphodiesterase-5 inhibitors (sildenafil, tadalafil, others), apomorphine (4 mg SL; side effect of vomiting diminishes with repeated use), intracavernosal treatment (PGE1, thymoxamine, others including papaverine), intraurethral (PGE1), vacuum devices and penile prostheses.
- For urinary tract dysfunction, treat infection. Consider the use of a regular voiding schedule and pelvic floor exercises for stress incontinence. Pharmacotherapy may include parasympathomimetics and α-adrenergic blockade to relieve sphincter hypertonicity. End-stage dysfunction may require intermittent self-catheterization.
- For patients with hypohidrosis or anhidrosis, advise caution about heat exposure. Moisturizers may be applied to dry feet and hands.
- Preventing hypoglycemia improves hypoglycemic unawareness.
- References (38,93).

14

Dementia and cerebral microvascular disease

Recent work has identified an important link between diabetes mellitus and the development of dementia. This connection requires attention and further research, potentially posing a major health burden on society.

KEY POINTS

- Persons with diabetes are at increased risk for both vascular cognitive impairment and for Alzheimer's disease (AD).
- Persons with diabetes are at increased risk for cerebral microvascular disease that leads to covert brain infarction and white matter lesions.
- Treatment for cognitive impairment and dementia may include acetylcholinesterase inhibitors or memantine, pharmacological and behavioral therapy for neuropsychiatric complications, assistance with activities of daily living, and caregiver support.
- It is currently not known whether careful control of vascular risk factors or mental or physical exercise prevents dementia or slows its course.
- It is currently not known whether more strict control of hyperglycemia prevents diabetic cerebral microvascular disease or dementia.

DEFINITIONS

- Dementia may be defined as (based on *DSM-IV* criteria) (*i*) cognitive impairment in memory and at least one other domain (e.g., executive function, visuospatial function, or language), (*ii*) impairment sufficient to cause a significant decline in social or occupational functioning, and (*iii*) impairment not occurring exclusively during an episode of delirium.

- Mild cognitive impairment defines an intermediate state between normal and demented, characterized by (*i*) cognitive symptoms, (*ii*) essentially preserved social and other functioning, and (*iii*) objective evidence of poor cognitive performance on testing (94).
  - Poor cognitive performance is based on standardized neuropsychological testing that is less than 1 to 1.5 standard deviations below average for age and education.

CLINICAL FEATURES

- See chapter 2 and chapter 3, section "Dementia in a Diabetic Patient."

DIAGNOSIS

- Dementia is a clinical diagnosis and is made based on history and mental status examination, and is not based solely on performance below a cutoff on a cognitive test.
- Diagnosis may be aided by objective testing of cognitive performance as provided by neuropsychological testing.
- Brief global assessments of cognitive function are available. The most widely used are the Mini-Mental Status Examination (MMSE) and the Montreal Cognitive Assessment Tool (MoCA).
  - The MMSE ranges from 0 to 30, with most points assigned for memory and orientation.
    - A score below 24 often indicates dementia.
  - The MoCA (authors' preference; see Table 2.3) also ranges from 0 to 30 (http://www.mocatest.org/).
    - It is more sensitive to mild degrees of impairment than the MMSE.
    - It includes more tests of working memory and executive function and therefore may be more sensitive to non-Alzheimer's causes of dementia. This requires validation.
    - A cutoff of <26 suggests the presence of either MCI (mild cognitive impairment) or dementia, but there is substantial overlap in scores between those with MCI and dementia.

ETIOLOGY

- A multitude of neurological and systemic diseases can cause dementia. Table 14.1 provides a list of the most important or potentially reversible causes.
- A limited subset is responsible for most cases identified in routine practice. Recent research suggests dementias are frequently linked to more than one type of neuropathology in the same brain (95).

Table 14.1 Select Causes of Dementia or Dementia Mimics, Emphasizing Common or Treatable Disorders

Neurodegenerative causes
    AD
    Lewy body disease
    Frontotemporal dementia and its variants
    Corticobasal syndrome
    Progressive supranuclear palsy
    Huntington's disease
    Parkinson's disease
Cerebrovascular diseases
    Cerebral infarction
    Cerebral hemorrhage
Other brain structural causes
    Hydrocephalus, including normal pressure hydrocephalus
    Subdural hematoma
    Brain tumor
Infectious causes
    HIV dementia complex
    Creutzfeldt–Jakob disease and other prion diseases
    Progressive multifocal leukoencephalopathy
Inflammatory causes
    Multiple sclerosis
    Vasculitis
    Nonvasculitis autoimmune inflammatory meningoencephalopathies (NAIM)
    Paraneoplastic disoders (including limbic encephalitis)
Metabolic or endocrine causes
    Hypothyroidism or hyperthyroidism
    Cortisol deficiency
    Vitamin B12 deficiency
    Other nutritional causes (e.g., thiamine or niacin deficiency)
    Ethanol abuse
    Hepatic encephalopathy
    Encephalopathy associated with renal disease
Iatrogenic causes
    Sedative medications
    Neuroleptics
Psychiatric diseases
    Depression ("pseudodementia")
    Schizophrenia or associated disorders
    Bipolar disorder

- AD and cerebrovascular disease are the most commonly found pathologies and are frequently present in the same brain (95).
- Vascular dementia may result from (*i*) multiple infarctions (known as multi-infarct dementia) or multiple hemorrhages, (*ii*) strategic infarct or

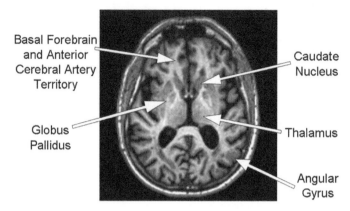

Basal Forebrain
and Anterior
Cerebral Artery
Territory

Caudate
Nucleus

Globus
Pallidus

Thalamus

Angular
Gyrus

Other strategic locations include: genu of the internal
capsule, corpus callosum, medial temporal lobe

Figure 14.1   Strategic locations for cerebral infarction in diabetic patients.

hemorrhage in a single brain region critical for cognitive function
(Fig. 14.1) or (*iii*) subcortical ischemic lesions (white matter lesions or
small subcortical infarctions) (Fig. 14.2).

EPIDEMIOLOGY AND RISK FACTORS

- The lifetime cumulative risk in persons aged 65 years is 1 in 10 men and 1
  in 5 women according to the Framingham study (96).
- The incidence and prevalence are highly age dependent (Table 14.2).
- The prevalence of mild cognitive impairment is not well defined but is
  approximately equal to or greater than the prevalence of dementia for each
  age stratum.
- Risk factors for dementia have been clarified in large population-based
  studies. These risk factors have also been associated with the clinical
  diagnosis of AD, the most common pathology associated with dementia.
- Diabetes increases the risk of vascular dementia by approximately 2.0- to
  3.0-fold (97) and the risk of Alzheimer's dementia by 1.5-fold (98).
  - Studies are primarily limited to type 2 diabetes.
  - There is limited information on the risk in type 1 diabetes, although
    decreased cognitive performance in type 1 diabetes has been demon-
    strated compared with controls.

SPECIAL CONSIDERATIONS IN DIABETES

- Persons with diabetes are at increased risk for both vascular cognitive
  impairment and AD.

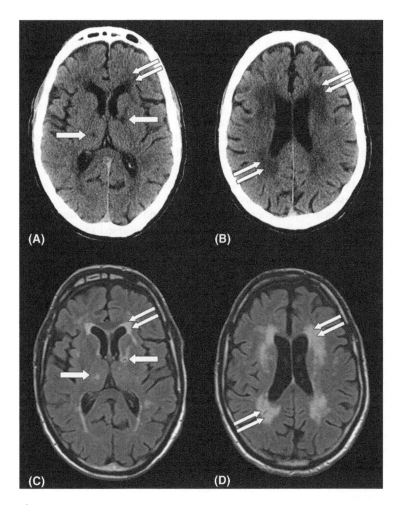

Figure 14.2 Microvascular disease of the brain. A lacunar infarct is demonstrated on CT (**A**) and MRI fluid attenuated inversion recovery (FLAIR) sequence (**B**). White matter lesions, also known as leukoaraiosis, are seen as hypodensity on CT (**C**) and hyperintensity on T2-weighted MRI sequences, such as this FLAIR sequence (**D**). The wide arrows indicate lacunar infarcts and the narrow arrows white matter abnormalities.

Table 14.2 Prevalence of Dementia by Age Category

Age	Dementia (all causes) (%)	Probable AD (%)
≤70	<5	<2
71–79	5	2
80–89	24	18
≥90	37	30

Estimates are from a U.S. population-based study.
Source: From Ref. 110.

- Vascular cognitive impairment in diabetes may result from (*i*) cardioembolic ischemic stroke as a result of accelerated coronary artery atherosclerosis with ischemic cardiomyopathy, (*ii*) large artery ischemic stroke as a result of accelerated atherosclerosis of the cervical and intracranial large arteries (cerebral macrovascular disease), or (*iii*) diabetic microvascular disease of the cerebral circulation, resulting in white matter lesions and small subcortical infarctions.
- Diabetes causes microvascular disease through multiple mechanisms including hyperglycemia-induced glycosylation of proteins and increased superoxide production.
  - In the brain, this manifests as small subcortical infarctions and white matter lesions (leukoaraiosis).
  - Small subcortical infarctions are typically found in the brain stem, basal ganglia, thalamus, and white matter and are presumed to result from thrombotic vascular occlusion of small penetrating arteries (Fig. 14.2, panels A, B). These infarcts may be termed "covert" because, in most cases, they do not cause overt stroke symptoms but are instead associated with risk of cognitive impairment and cognitive decline.
  - White matter lesions are usually symmetric and found in the periventricular region or less commonly in the subcortical white matter (Fig. 14.2, panels C, D) (99). They are presumed to result from ischemic demyelination, although a role for increased blood-brain barrier permeability has also been proposed.
  - The presence of covert infarctions or severe white matter lesions increases the subsequent risk of dementia by 1.5- to 1.7-fold. Progression to dementia is often associated with new infarctions or progression of white matter lesions (100).
- There is an increased risk of AD in persons with diabetes.
  - The neuropathological hallmarks of AD are senile plaques, composed of β-amyloid and neurofibrillary tangles that consist of aggregated tau protein.
  - Current evidence suggests a critical role for β-amyloid in the pathogenesis.
    - β-Amyloid is an aggregate of Aβ peptide fragments generated by cleavage of the amyloid precursor protein.
  - The increased risk of AD in persons with diabetes could be explained by (*i*) an increased prevalence of covert brain infarctions and white matter lesions that decrease cognitive reserve and make the brain more vulnerable to Alzheimer pathology, (*ii*) deleterious effects of hyperglycemia on brain function that make the brain more vulnerable to Alzheimer pathology, or (*iii*) an acceleration of Alzheimer-type pathology in the setting of diabetes. There is insufficient evidence to determine to what extent these three hypotheses are correct (97).

- ○ Several intriguing observations support the connection between diabetes and incidence or acceleration of AD (101).
  - ▪ Hyperinsulinemia may increase cerebral Aβ production.
  - ▪ Hyperinsulinemia may decrease cerebral Aβ clearance by competing with Aβ for insulin-degrading enzyme, a protein that degrades both Aβ and insulin.
  - ▪ Brains of persons with diabetes are more likely to have Alzheimer pathology than controls (102).

PROGNOSIS

- • AD and other neurodegenerative diseases are slowly progressive.
- • Vascular cognitive impairment may have a more variable course.
  - ○ Cognitive impairment following stroke may be static.
  - ○ Cognitive impairment from cerebral microvascular disease may be relatively static, progressive, or stepwise progressive.

TREATMENT

- • Treatment guidelines are available (103–108).
- • Acetylcholinesterase inhibitors and memantine improve cognitive performance without affecting the underlying neurodegeneration (Table 14.3).
  - ○ Effects on quality of life are more controversial and appear to be relatively modest.
  - ○ Acetylcholinesterase inhibitors may cause bradycardia and should be used with caution in persons with cardiac conduction disorders.
  - ○ These drugs have been most frequently studied in AD.
  - ○ Several studies suggest benefit in vascular dementia or mixed dementia as well.
  - ○ A small study suggests benefit for Lewy body dementia.
- • Manage neurobehavioral complications of dementia, if present.
  - ○ Agitation, paranoia, or abulia may be seen particularly in the moderate-to-severe stages of dementia.
  - ○ Neuroleptics may have some role for controlling agitation but have been associated with increased mortality in randomized controlled trials (absolute risk increase in one meta-analysis was 1.9%, number needed to harm 53)(109). This is thought to be a class effect. Select patients may benefit from their judicious use if they provide improved quality of life and increased safety for the patient and caregiver.
- • Treat comorbid depression if present.
  - ○ Often presents in the earlier stages when insight is relatively preserved.
  - ○ True pseudodementia (that is, "dementia" that completely reverses with treatment of depression) is rare.

Table 14.3 Drugs for Cognition in Alzheimer's Disease

Medication	Action	Effective dose (mg)	Formulation	FDA indication
Donepezil	Acetycholinesterase inhibitor	5–10	Tablet or orally disintegrating tablet	Mild-to-severe AD
Galantamine	Acetycholinesterase inhibitor	8–24	Tablet, oral solution, or extended-release tablet	Mild-to-moderate AD
Rivastigmine	Acetycholinesterase inhibitor	6–12	Capsule, oral solution, or 24-hr extended-release patch	Mild-to-moderate AD
Memantine	NMDA receptor antagonist	20	Tablet or oral solution	Moderate-to-severe AD

Refer to the package labeling for detailed dosing information; several require initial dose titration to the effective dose. All have also been studied in randomized controlled trials for vascular dementia and mixed dementia with some evidence for benefit, but none have an approved U.S. FDA indication for these diseases. Rivastigmine was beneficial in a small study of patients with Lewy body disease and dementia.

Abbreviation: FDA, U.S. Food and Drug Administration.

- Identify and manage vascular risk factors.
- Assistance with instrumental and basic activities of daily living is necessary as the disease progresses.
- Support for caregivers with appropriate use of respite care, group therapy, and day programs are important.
- Make plans for how financial and other affairs will be handled if/when the capacity to make informed decisions is lost (e.g., by arrangements for legal guardianship or proxy).
- Information and support programs for patients and caregivers are available on the web through organizations such as the Alzheimer's Association (http://www.alz.org) and the Alzheimer's Society of Canada (http://www.alzheimer.ca).
- Evidence for the benefit of strict control of hyperglycemia to control or prevent cognitive impairment or dementia is inconclusive.
  - Randomized controlled trials of strict glucose control in type 2 diabetes have shown a reduction in microvascular disease in the retina and kidney, but without information on cerebral microvascular disease (an evaluation that requires brain MR studies).
  - Similarly, trials have to date not provided definitive information on whether more strict glucose control prevents dementia or alters the rate of change in cognitive performance on standardized testing.
- Reference (48).

15

Neurological infections in diabetes

Patients with diabetes mellitus are at risk for a number of serious infectious complications. While some involve direct infection of the CNS or PNS, others arise secondary to diabetic neurological complications.

KEY POINTS

- Patients with diabetes mellitus can be regarded as immunocompromised and prone to a number of infections, including neurological infections.
- Both humoral and cell-mediated immunity are impaired in diabetes; risks may be higher in older patients.
- Several uncommon infections are most frequently associated with diabetes mellitus, including mucormycosis, aspergillosis, spinal epidural abscess, and others.
- Severe forms of systemic infections including pneumonia or urinary tract infection can lead to altered mental status in diabetic patients and a deterioration in glucose control.
- Diabetic neurological complications such as urinary bladder stasis or foot insensitivity are risk factors for infection (urinary tract infections, osteomyelitis).

MUCORMYCOSIS (ZYGOMYCOSIS, PHYCOMYCOSIS, RHINOCEREBRAL MUCORMYCOSIS)

- Fungi of the order Mucorales: this infection complicates diabetic ketoacidosis or other conditions involving an immunocompromised host.
- Onset is a nasal turbinate and paranasal sinus infection with local spread.
- Symptoms include fever, headache, orbital and facial pain, orbital and facial swelling, and nasal congestion.

- Symptoms are proptosis, ophthalmoplegia, edema and eschar formation, altered level of consciousness, confusion, cerebral hemorrhagic infarction, loss of vision, and cavernous sinus syndrome.
- Diagnosis is by aseptate hyphae on histology or tissue culture.
- Prognosis is guarded.
- Preferred treatment is antifungal therapy (Amphotericin B or newer antifungal agents), treatment of ketoacidosis, and surgical debridement.
- Reference (111).

ASPERGILLOSIS

- *Aspergillus fumigatus* is a common resident of the environment and lodges in the upper respiratory tract; patients may have a "fungus ball" identified by chest radiography; it may also arise from the paranasal sinuses.
- Invasive aspergillosis is a multisystem disorder that develops in immuno-compromised hosts and has a high mortality rate.
- Invasive cerebral aspergillosis is a rare but life-threatening complication that spreads to brain from the blood stream.
- Aspergillosis is angioinvasive because it targets blood vessel wall elastin.
- Diabetic patients having undergone kidney or pancreas transplantation are at risk for its development, but there are also rare reports in diabetes alone.
- Clinical presentations include headache accompanied by multiple cranial nerve palsies, decreased LOC, seizures and focal neurological signs and symptoms.
- Angioinvasive aspergillosis may present with cerebral infarction that later evolves into single or multiple cerebral abscess; *Aspergillus* may also be associated with a fungal meningitis.
- References (112,113).

SPINAL EPIDURAL ABSCESS

- A neurosurgical emergency.
- More common in patients with diabetes mellitus and in immunocompro-mised individuals.
- Epidural catheters, spinal surgery, skin abscesses, and furuncles can be the source of the infection, often from *Staphylococcus aureus.*
- Presents with fever, back pain, symptoms of nerve root irritation, and myelopathy (sensory level, lower limb weakness, spasticity, upgoing toes and brisk reflexes, sphincter dysfunction).
- Diagnosis is by spinal MR imaging; thoracic lesions are the most common site of involvement.
- Treatment of choice is laminectomy and antibiotics.
- Reference (114).

OTHER UNCOMMON CNS INFECTIONS

- *Chryseobacterium indologenes* bacteremia and decreased LOC following ketoacidosis and cerebral edema.
- Malignant otitis externa: a severe *Pseudomonas aeruginosa* infection of the external ear that may be associated with involvement of the seventh cranial nerve, other cranial nerves, meninges, sigmoid sinus—MRI with gadolinium is the preferred imaging modality; treatment is debridement and antibiotics.
- Reactivation of tuberculosis can occur in patients with diabetes.
- References (111,115).

DIAGNOSIS AND MANAGEMENT OF BACTERIAL MENINGITIS

- Bacterial meningitis is a medical emergency, and treatment should not be delayed by diagnostic measures.
- Symptoms are new headache, neck stiffness, fever, rash, decreased LOC, and occasionally focal neurological symptoms.
- Immediate lumbar puncture is required if there are no focal findings, seizures, or decreased LOC: RBC, WBC count (with differential), protein, glucose, gram stain, and culture. Typical findings are CSF neutrophilic pleocytosis, low glucose, and elevated protein.
- CT scan, if immediately available, can precede lumbar puncture if there are focal neurological findings, seizures, or decreased level of consciousness.
- Blood cultures, concurrent serum glucose should be drawn together with lumbar puncture.
- Empirical therapy (before culture results) given IV: third generation cephalosporin (e.g., ceftriaxone 2 g q12h) AND vancomycin (1 g q8–12h); Add ampicillin for poorly controlled diabetics or those with end-organ complications (2 g q4h).
- Dexamethasone 10 mg IV q6h for four days may reduce long-term sequelae in patients with pneumococcal meningitis, but can also worsen hyperglycemia (see chap. 4).

FOOT INFECTIONS IN PATIENTS WITH DIABETIC NEUROPATHY

- The risk factors for foot infection are similar to those causing ulceration: abrasions, blistering, and penetrating trauma.
- Insensitivity to injury and poor healing from sensory polyneuropathy and foot deformity from muscle denervation (neuropathy involving motor axons) predispose to ulceration.
- Foot infections are often associated with *S. aureus* or β-hemolytic streptococcus; severe, chronic, or previously treated infections are often polymicrobial.

- There is a high risk of associated foot ulceration and osteomyelitis requiring amputation.
- Not all ulcers require antibiotic therapy; results of culture swabs may be unreliable.
- Infections include cellulitis, myositis, osteomyelitis, abscesses, necrotizing fasciitis, tendinitis, and septic arthritis.
- Infection typically is suggested by purulent discharge, foul odor, erythema, and swelling. Note that pain can be absent and that systemic signs of infection are uncommon unless the infection is severe and deep seated.
- Features that suggest osteomyelitis: swollen red ("sausage") toe, elevated ESR (>70 mm), visible bone or palpable bone on palpating the wound, nonhealing ulcer, unexplained leukocytosis, radiological evidence of underlying bone destruction, ulcerated area greater than 2 cm^2 or 3-mm deep.
- Imaging by plain radiographs detects foreign bodies and tissue gas; earlier diagnosis of osteomyelitis requires nuclear imaging using technetium, gallium or a white blood cell scan (or a combination of these) or bone MR.
- Aggressive surgical debridement and antibiotic therapy are usually required for foot infections. Complete healing requires off-loading, cessation of smoking, treatment of edema and follow-up studies such as repeat imaging.
- Reference (116).

URINARY TRACT INFECTIONS IN DIABETES MELLITUS

- There may be a higher prevalence in older diabetic patients.
- Bladder overfilling and stasis are probable risk factors.
- Complications include bacteriuria, lower urinary tract infections with atypical symptoms (e.g., confusion), emphysematous cystitis, pyelonephritis, and perinephric abscess.
- Reference (111).

HERPES ZOSTER IN DIABETES MELLITUS

- Herpes zoster arises from reactivation of varicella infection in childhood.
- Presents with prodromal pain followed by painful red vesicular rash, then crusting and healing in one or more skin dermatomal distributions, especially the trunk; overall course of the skin disease is over 7 to 14 days.
- Increased prevalence is noted in elderly and immunosuppressed patients.
- It is uncertain if the prevalence is higher with diabetes mellitus alone, but an increased prevalence in diabetic patients undergoing pancreatic transplantation has been confirmed.
- Postherpetic neuralgia is a common and severe cause of neuropathic pain and develops in 30% of cases of zoster (higher in older individuals).
- Herpes zoster ophthalmicus involving the first trigeminal nerve territory (forehead, eye) is a serious risk factor for eye damage.

- Other complications of herpes zoster include motor and sensory nerve root damage, transverse myelitis, meningoencephalitis, CNS vasculitis, Ramsay Hunt syndrome (7th cranial neuropathy, see chap. 11).
- Diagnostic confusion with truncal radiculopathy may occur (see chap. 11).
- May be prevented by vaccination.

OTHER INFECTIONS IN DIABETES MELLITUS

- Fungal nail infections of toes (onychomycosis); mucocutaneous candidiasis
- Pneumonia, cellulitis, and necrotizing fasciitis
- Periodontal disease
- General increased risk of hospital-acquired infection
- Reference (117).

16

Neurological complications of diabetic nephropathy

Diabetic nephropathy is among the triad of serious complications of diabetes mellitus (neuropathy, nephropathy, and retinopathy) and is the most common cause of acquired renal failure. Diabetic patients with renal failure on dialysis are at risk for developing several associated neurological problems.

KEY POINTS

- Uremia may be associated with encephalopathy, polyneuropathy, focal neuropathies (mononeuropathies), and accelerated atherosclerosis.
- Patients with renal transplants are at risk for immunosuppressive complications.

UREMIC POLYNEUROPATHY

- Risk of uremic polyneuropathy increases as serum creatinine rises above 450 μmol/L (5.0 mg%).
- Older literature suggests a prevalence of 50% to 60% of polyneuropathy in dialysis patients and higher if nerve conduction studies are used to identify it.
- Risk of uremic polyneuropathy in the last decade may be reduced by the use of erythropoietin or other factors, but definitive studies on prevalence are unavailable.
- Symptoms include restless legs, paresthesia, weakness, cramps, dysesthesia, burning or electric sensations, tightness, paradoxical thermal sensation (cold misinterpreted as heat).
- Signs of polyneuropathy include loss of light touch, pinprick, temperature and vibration sensations, loss of deep tendon reflexes, atrophy, and weakness.

- Some cases have been rapidly progressive, associated with quadriparesis; others with a subacute course and prominent demyelination; patients with subacute disease have responded to high-flux hemodialysis.
- Prominent burning sensations may suggest a superimposed B vitamin deficiency.
- Sural nerve conduction is a sensitive index of early uremic neuropathy, and peroneal motor conduction velocity is an accurate index of its severity or response to transplantation.
- Findings of primary demyelination (prominent conduction velocity slowing) and axon loss (loss of motor and sensory potentials) are identified on nerve conduction studies.
- EMG signs of denervation (fibrillation potentials, positive sharp waves) may be less evident in patients with renal failure and diabetes (118,119).
- There is no evidence that more intensive renal dialysis is useful for most types of uremic polyneuropathy, but renal transplantation appears to reverse the condition.

MONONEUROPATHIES ASSOCIATED WITH RENAL FAILURE

- Carpal tunnel syndrome is prominent in renal failure, possibly linked to β2-microglobulin/amyloid deposition in the carpal tunnel (see chap. 10).
- Ulnar neuropathy at the elbow and peroneal neuropathy at the fibular head from entrapment may be prominent in bedridden patients.
- Ischemic forearm neuropathy may develop as a complication of the placement of vascular grafts for hemodialysis: symptoms are pain, paresthesia, sensory loss, and weakness in the median, ulnar, or radial nerve territories; neuropathy is secondary to ischemia from shunting of arterial blood flow away from the forearm nerve trunks; recovery may occur if the shunt is revised (120).
- Coagulopathy of renal failure can rarely be associated with retroperitoneal hemorrhage and compression of the lumbosacral plexus.

UREMIC ENCEPHALOPATHY

- Uremic encephalopathy is associated with hyperventilation from metabolic acidosis, myoclonus, and seizures.
- Develops more rapidly if the onset of renal failure is acute.
- The spectrum of encephalopathy ranges from mild cognitive dysfunction to coma.
- Features of acute uremic encephalopathy include lethargy, irritability, confusion, disorientation, dysarthria, tremor, myoclonus, asterixis, tetany, and fluctuating hemiparesis.
- Seizures can be focal or generalized.
- Toxicity from retained medications that are renally excreted may cause encephalopathy (e.g., seizures from penicillin toxicity).
- Uremic encephalopathy is reversible with dialysis.

- Encephalopathy with chronic renal failure may be more insidious: lethargy, fatigue, headaches, depression, irritability and restlessness, poor concentration, sleep disturbance, seizures (focal or generalized), intention or multifocal myoclonus, mild dysarthria, and postural action tremor.
- EEG abnormalities are encountered in chronic uremic encephalopathy: generalized slowing, slow wave bursts, triphasic waves, prominent response to photic stimulation (photomyogenic response), and epileptiform potentials.

HYPERTENSIVE ENCEPHALOPATHY AND POSTERIOR REVERSIBLE ENCEPHALOPATHY SYNDROME

- Hypertensive encephalopathy and *p*osterior *r*eversible *e*ncephalopathy *s*yndrome (PRES) are overlapping disorders; a hallmark of hypertensive encephalopathy has been the presence of altered mental status and papilledema.
- A medical and neurological emergency.
- Symptoms include headache, lethargy, confusion, visual disturbance, and seizures; cognitive changes range from somnolence to coma; visual disturbances include hemianopsia, cortical blindness, and visual neglect.
- Brain imaging studies typically show parietal-occipital hemispheric white matter abnormalities, but other areas of the CNS and gray matter may also be involved; abnormalities may be prominent on diffusion-weighted images.
- Immunosuppressive agents used for transplantation are an important risk factor for the development of PRES.
- Effects of hypertension and diabetes may be additive in causing damage to the microvascular endothelium of the brain.

OTHER NEUROLOGICAL COMPLICATIONS

- Confusion may be associated with peritonitis in patients undergoing peritoneal dialysis.
- Subdural hematoma is reported in 1% to 3% of dialysis patients in the older literature, especially if the patient is also anticoagulated; there may be no history of head trauma. It presents with headache, confusion, focal neurological signs, and gait disturbance (apraxia of gait).
- Complications of renal transplantation: opportunistic infections, complications of glucocorticoids (encephalopathy, myopathy, others), and other antirejection therapies (e.g., tremor secondary to cyclosporine).
- Dialysis disequilibrium syndrome may occur from a rapid osmotic shift with treatment: headache, restlessness or somnolence, GI upset, cognitive changes, asterixis, and myoclonus; onset during or just after hemodialysis.

References (121–126).

17

Uncommon neurological disorders associated with diabetes

Diabetes mellitus may be an important feature of a number of other multisystem disorders. Several have concurrent neurological involvement as a primary or secondary feature. The list of these uncommon conditions continues to grow.

KEY POINTS

- Several primary neurological disorders may also be associated with diabetes mellitus.
- In most instances, management does not differ from patients with uncomplicated diabetes mellitus. An exception is that greater attention should be applied toward avoiding hypoglycemia in patients with associated seizure disorders since it may lower the seizure threshold.
- Consider mitochondrial disease in patients with a strong maternal inheritance of type 2 diabetes, short stature, and hearing loss; manifestations include neuropathy, myopathy, encephalopathy, stroke-like episodes, seizures, or migraines.
- Avoid metformin in patients with suspected mitochondrial diseases because of the risk of lactic acidosis.

WOLFRAM SYNDROME

- Wolfram syndrome is a rare multisystem autosomal recessive neurodegenerative disorder.
- It is also known as DIDMOAD (diabetes insipidus, diabetes mellitus, optic atrophy, and deafness).
- The condition is secondary to a mutation of the WFS1 gene on chromosome 4 (wolframin is the gene product).

- It involves <1% of patients with type 1 juvenile onset diabetes mellitus.
- Early death occurs before the age of 50.
- Reported neurological features include optic atrophy, mental retardation, seizures, hearing loss (especially high tone), nystagmus, depression, psychosis, ataxia, peripheral neuropathy, dementia, neurogenic respiratory failure, startle myoclonus, axial rigidity, and Parinaud syndrome; Parinaud syndrome involves paralysis of upgaze that may accompany convergence-retraction nystagmus, conjugate downgaze, eyelid retraction, and loss of pupil accommodation to near vision.
- Pathological findings are atrophy of brain stem and cerebellum with multifocal loss of neurons.
- Other problems include renal tract abnormalities and gonadal disorders.
- References (126,127).

MITOCHONDRIAL DISORDERS

- Several types exist depending on the mutation in nuclear or mitochondrial DNA and how many abnormal mitochondria are in a given tissue (heteroplasmy).
- Classical phenotypes may only be partially expressed (oligosymptomatic).
- Mitochondrial disorders are frequently maternally inherited and involve a large number of mutations.
- The disorder MELAS, refers to mitochondrial encephalopathy, lactic acidosis, and stroke-like episodes, is one of the classical phenotypes that has been extensively described (most common mutation is an A–G transition mutation at position 3243 of the mitochondrial genome).
- Manifestations of MELAS are seizures, encephalopathy, stroke-like episodes, short stature, cognitive dysfunction, migraine headaches, depression, hearing loss, cardiomyopathy and cardiac conduction deficits, myopathy, and neuropathy.
- Type 2 diabetes mellitus is identified in 33%; some cohorts have had diabetes in all carriers by age 70.
- Avoid use of metformin because of the risk of lactic acidosis in these patients.
- Peripheral neuropathy is present in 22% of these cases and may be mistaken for diabetic polyneuropathy.
- Consider mitochondrial disease in the presence of a strong, matrilineal clustering of diabetes, presence of short stature, and hearing loss.
- Gastrointestinal manifestations may be prominent and erroneously attributed to diabetic autonomic neuropathy—constipation, gastric discomfort, others.
- Other mitochondrial syndromes (uncommon): MERRF (myoclonic epilepsy with ragged red fibers), Pearson syndrome, Wolfram syndrome (see earlier), Leigh disease, CPEO (chronic progressive external ophthalmoplegia), NARP (neuropathy, ataxia, and retinitis pigmentosa), and LHON (Leber hereditary optic neuropathy), CADN (cerebellar ataxia, deafness, and narcolepsy),

Feigenbaum syndrome (cognitive dysfunction, deafness, atherosclerosis, other deficits).
- References (128,129).

MYOTONIC DYSTROPHY TYPE I

- Myotonic dystrophy type 1 (DM1) is an autosomal dominant muscular dystrophy secondary to CTG triplet expansion.
- Features are progressive muscle weakness, frontal balding, temporal muscle atrophy, myotonia of muscles, cataracts, hypogonadism, cognitive dysfunction, and deficits of arousal.
- DM1 patients may have diabetes mellitus, but it is not clearly secondary to insulin resistance; proinsulin levels are elevated.
- References (129,130).

ACROMEGALY

- Acromegaly arises from a pituitary tumor secreting GH (growth hormone).
- Its features include enlargement of hands and feet, head and face with deepening of voice, skull, mandibular, and tongue enlargement.
- Pituitary tumor enlargement may be associated with headache and visual loss; bitemporal field deficit is the classical early visual deficit.
- The prevalence of diabetes mellitus in acromegaly is reported to be between 19% and 56%.
- Insulin resistance is linked to elevated GH levels.
- Rarely acromegaly is associated with ketoacidosis.
- Reference (131).

MUSCLE INFARCTION

- Muscle infarction is a rare condition reported in diabetic adults.
- Sudden pain, swelling in one thigh, may recur on the contralateral side; elevated serum CK level.
- Diagnosis may be made on muscle CT or MR imaging studies.
- Important to exclude a systemic embolization syndrome (e.g., from a cardiac source).
- Specific therapy is not available and slow recovery is expected.

FRIEDREICH'S ATAXIA

- Friedreich's ataxia is an autosomal recessive neurodegenerative disorder associated with diabetes mellitus.
- Symptoms include progressive ataxia, dysarthria, square wave ocular jerks, loss of reflexes, loss of vibration sense, upper motor neuron weakness and spasticity, pes cavus, hearing loss, and cardiomyopathy.
- The onset occurs in childhood with a life expectancy of <50 years.

- Associated with a GAA-triplet expansion in the frataxin gene.
- More prevalent in Europe, Middle East, North Africa, and India.
- Electrophysiology shows signs of sensory axonal neuropathy.
- Frequent requirement for insulin in longer-standing disease.
- Reference (132).

POEMS SYNDROME (CROW–FUKASE SYNDROME)

- POEMS syndrome is a multisystem disorder with the cardinal features of: *P*olyneuropathy, *O*rganomegaly, *E*ndocrinopathy, *M* protein, and *S*kin changes.
- Polyneuropathy in POEMS syndrome differs from diabetic polyneuropathy by exhibiting more prominent features of primary demyelination resembling chronic inflammatory demyelinating polyneuropathy (CIDP).
- Organomegaly includes splenomegaly, hepatomegaly, lymphadenopathy.
- Endocrinopathy includes abnormalities adrenal, thyroid, pituitary, gonadal, parathyroid, and pancreatic function; 54% have multiple endocrinopathies.
- M protein refers to a clonal plasma proliferative disorder usually lambda subtype, with osteosclerotic myeloma or Castleman's disease (angiofollicular lymph node hyperplasia)
- Skin changes include hyperpigmentation, hypertrichosis, plethora, hemangiomata, white nails, edema, clubbing.
- Papilledema, thrombocytosis, polycythemia, weight loss, ascites, and pleural effusion and others are additional features.
- Abnormalities in glucose metabolism are identified in 48% of POEMs patients and frank diabetes mellitus is present in 16%.
- Reference (133).

WILLIAMS–BEUREN SYNDROME

- Williams–Beuren syndrome arises from a spontaneous mutation during gamete formation causing a deletion of 26 to 28 genes. It is a multisystem disorder.
- Features are abnormal facial structure, stenosis of medium and large arteries from smooth muscle overgrowth, myxomatous cardiac valvular degeneration, hypertension, glucose intolerance or diabetes (75% of patients), hypercalcemia, short stature, joint laxity, abnormal personality and psychiatric disorders, premature aging, developmental delay, and others.
- Neurological problems are sensorineural high-tone hearing loss, cerebral infarction, cognitive dysfunction, hypotonia, hyperreflexia, cerebellar dysfunction, and type I Chiari malformation. Cerebral atrophy is present on imaging studies.
- Reference (134).

ALSTROM SYNDROME (ALMS)

- ALMS is an autosomal recessive syndrome with obesity, retinitis pigmentosa, deafness, and diabetes mellitus.
- Other features: insulin resistance, hypertension, hyperlipidemia, hyperuricemia, dilated cardiomyopathy, chronic active hepatitis, acanthosis nigrans.
- Reference (129).

ACERULOPLASMINEMIA

- Aceruloplasminemia is an autosomal recessive disorder from a deficiency in ceruloplasmin leading to basal ganglia overload.
- Features include cerebellar ataxia, dementia, extrapyramidal findings, and diabetes mellitus.
- Reference (129).

ATAXIA-TELANGIECTASIA (LOUIS-BAR SYNDROME)

- Ataxia-telangiectasisa is an autosomal recessive involving a mutation of the ATM protein that is required for DNA repair.
- Its features are ataxia, telangiectasias, type 2 DM with insulin resistance, increased risk of malignancies, immune compromise.
- Reference (129).

KLINEFELTER'S SYNDROME

- Klinefelter's syndrome is caused by an additional X chromosome in males.
- Features are a tall, slender body with hypogonadism, gynecomastia, and osteoporosis.
- Neurological features include seizures, motor delay, speech, attention, learning and reading deficits, and behavioral difficulties.
- Associated with autoimmune type 1 diabetes mellitus.
- References (135,136).

OTHER NEURODEGENERATIVE DISORDERS LINKED WITH DIABETES MELLITUS

- Alzheimer's dementia (associated with type 2 diabetes mellitus).
- Down's syndrome (associated with both type 1 and type 2 diabetes mellitus).
- Parkinson's disease (impaired glucose tolerance)
- Huntington's disease.
- Bardet–Biedl syndrome (autosomal recessive, polydactyly, mental retardation, pigmentary retinopathy, renal dysplasia, hepatic fibrosis, obesity, hypogonadism).

- Narcolepsy.
- Stiff-person syndrome (SPS; associated with type 1 DM, anti-GAD antibodies and treated with benzodiazepines; other variants also reported)
- Prader–Willi syndrome (mental retardation, hypotonia, other deficits).
- Thiamine responsive megaloblastic anemia syndrome.
- Turner syndrome (loss of a sex chromosome; includes mental retardation, nystagmus, strabismus, sexual immaturity, and other deficits).
- Spinocerebellar ataxia (SCA) types 3 and 6.
- Werner syndrome (premature aging).
- Herrmann syndrome (ataxia and epilepsy).
- Reference (129).

References

1. American Diabetes Association. Diagnosis and classification of diabetes mellitus. Diabetes Care 2010; 33(suppl 1):S62–S69.
2. Canadian Diabetes Association Clinical Practice Guidelines Expert Committee. Definition, Classification and Diagnosis of Diabetes and Other Dysglycemic Categories. 32nd ed. 2008:S10–S13.
3. Lyon AW, Larsen ET, Edwards AL. The impact of new guidelines for glucose tolerance testing on clinical practice and laboratory services. CMAJ 2004; 171:1067–1069.
4. Diabetes Control & Complications Trial Research Group. The effect of intensive treatment of diabetes on the development and progression of long-term complications in insulin-dependent diabetes mellitus. N Engl J Med 1993; 329:977–986.
5. National Institute for Health and Clinical Excellence. Type 2 Diabetes: Newer Agents, 2010.
6. IDF Clinical Guidelines Taskforce. Global Guideline for type 2 Diabetes, 2005.
7. Effect of intensive blood-glucose control with metformin on complications in overweight patients with type 2 diabetes (UKPDS 34). UK Prospective Diabetes Study (UKPDS) Group. Lancet 1998; 352:854–865.
8. Chiasson JL, Josse RG, Gomis R, et al. Acarbose for prevention of type 2 diabetes mellitus: the STOP-NIDDM randomised trial. Lancet 2002; 359:2072–2077.
9. Gerstein HC, Yusuf S, Bosch J, et al. Effect of rosiglitazone on the frequency of diabetes in patients with impaired glucose tolerance or impaired fasting glucose: a randomised controlled trial. Lancet 2006; 368:1096–1105.
10. Nissen SE, Wolski K. Effect of rosiglitazone on the risk of myocardial infarction and death from cardiovascular causes. N Engl J Med 2007; 356:2457–2471.
11. Patel A, MacMahon S, Chalmers J, et al. Intensive blood glucose control and vascular outcomes in patients with type 2 diabetes. N Engl J Med 2008; 358:2560–2572.
12. Duckworth W, Abraira C, Moritz T, et al. Glucose control and vascular complications in veterans with type 2 diabetes. N Engl J Med 2009; 360:129–139.

13. Gerstein HC, Miller ME, Byington RP, et al. Effects of intensive glucose lowering in type 2 diabetes. N Engl J Med 2008; 358:2545–2559.
14. Hirsch IB. Sliding scale insulin—time to stop sliding. JAMA 2009; 301:213–214.
15. Finfer S, Chittock DR, Su SY, et al. Intensive versus conventional glucose control in critically ill patients. N Engl J Med 2009; 360:1283–1297.
16. Ross RT. How to Examine the Nervous System. 4th ed. Totowa, NJ: Humana Press, 2006.
17. Mayo Clinic. Mayo Clinic Examinations in Neurology. 7th ed. Philadelphia: Mosby, 1997.
18. Theriault M, Dort J, Sutherland G, et al. A prospective quantitative study of sensory deficits after whole sural nerve biopsies in diabetic and nondiabetic patients. Surgical approach and the role of collateral sprouting. Neurology 1998; 50:480–484.
19. Suarez GA, Dyck PJ. Quantitative sensory assesment. In: Dyck PJ, Thomas PK, eds. Diabetic Neuropathy. 2nd ed. Philadelphia: W.B. Saunders, 2006:151–170.
20. Dyck PJ, Dyck PJ, Larson TS, et al. Patterns of quantitative sensation testing of hypoesthesia and hyperalgesia are predictive of diabetic polyneuropathy: a study of three cohorts. Nerve growth factor study group. Diabetes Care 2000; 23:510–517.
21. Lauria G, Cornblath DR, Johansson O, et al. EFNS guidelines on the use of skin biopsy in the diagnosis of peripheral neuropathy. Eur J Neurol 2005; 12:747–758.
22. Malik RA, Kallinikos P, Abbott CA, et al. Corneal confocal microscopy: a non-invasive surrogate of nerve fibre damage and repair in diabetic patients. Diabetologia 2003; 46:683–688.
23. Freeman R. Autonomic testing. In: Bolton CF, Brown WF, Aminoff M, eds. Neuromuscular Function and Disease. Toronto: W.B. Saunders, 2002:483–500.
24. Wasterlain CG, Chen JW. Mechanistic and pharmacologic aspects of status epilepticus and its treatment with new antiepileptic drugs. Epilepsia 2008; 49(suppl 9):63–73.
25. Elger CE, Schmidt D. Modern management of epilepsy: a practical approach. Epilepsy Behav 2008; 12:501–539.
26. Faught E. Monotherapy in adults and elderly persons. Neurology 2007; 69:S3–S9.
27. Schmidt D. Drug treatment of epilepsy: options and limitations. Epilepsy Behav 2009; 15:56–65.
28. Stephen LJ, Brodie MJ. Selection of antiepileptic drugs in adults. Neurol Clin 2009; 27:967–992.
29. Anonymous. Drugs for epilepsy, treatment guidelines. Med Lett Drugs Ther 2008; 6:37–46.
30. Pucelikova T, Dangas G, Mehran R. Contrast-induced nephropathy. Catheter Cardiovasc Interv 2008; 71:62–72.
31. Barrett BJ, Parfrey PS. Clinical practice. Preventing nephropathy induced by contrast medium. N Engl J Med 2006; 354:379–386.
32. Farmer A, Wade A, Goyder E, et al. Impact of self monitoring of blood glucose in the management of patients with non-insulin treated diabetes: open parallel group randomised trial. BMJ 2007; 335:132.
33. Davidson MB, Castellanos M, Kain D, et al. The effect of self monitoring of blood glucose concentrations on glycated hemoglobin levels in diabetic patients not taking insulin: a blinded, randomized trial. Am J Med 2005; 118:422–425.
34. Hypoglycemia in the Diabetes Control and Complications Trial. The Diabetes Control and Complications Trial Research Group. Diabetes 1997; 46:271–286.

35. Braithwaite SS, Barr WG, Rahman A, et al. Managing diabetes during glucocorticoid therapy. How to avoid metabolic emergencies. Postgrad Med 1998; 104:163–166.
36. Uzu T, Harada T, Sakaguchi M, et al. Glucocorticoid-induced diabetes mellitus: prevalence and risk factors in primary renal diseases. Nephron Clin Pract 2007; 105:c54–c57.
37. Iwamoto T, Kagawa Y, Naito Y, et al. Steroid-induced diabetes mellitus and related risk factors in patients with neurologic diseases. Pharmacotherapy 2004; 24:508–514.
38. Gries FA, Cameron NE, Low PA, et al. Textbook of Diabetic Neuropathy. New York: Thieme, 2003.
39. Freeby M, Ebner S. Ketoacidosis and hyperglycemic hyperosmolar state. Diabetes and the Brain. New York: Humana Press, 2009:159–182.
40. Young GB, Ropper AH, Bolton CF. Coma and Impaired Consciousness. Toronto: McGraw-Hill, 1998.
41. Moien-Afshari F, Tellez-Zenteno JF. Occipital seizures induced by hyperglycemia: a case report and review of literature. Seizure 2009; 18:382–385.
42. Tesfaye S, Kempler P. Painful diabetic neuropathy. Diabetologia 2005; 48:805–807.
43. Boulton AJ, Vinik AI, Arezzo JC, et al. Diabetic neuropathies: a statement by the American Diabetes Association. Diabetes Care 2005; 28:956–962.
44. Boulton AJM. Treatment of painful diabetic neuropathy. In: Malik RA, Veves A, eds. Diabetic Neuropathy, Clinical Management. 2nd ed. Totowa: Humana Press, 2007:351–365.
45. Frier BM. Hypoglycemia. In: Biessels GJ, Luchsinger JA, eds. Diabetes and the Brain. New York: Humana, 2010:131–157.
46. Hankey GJ, Eikelboom JW. Adding aspirin to clopidogrel after TIA and ischemic stroke: benefits do not match risks. Neurology 2005; 64:1117–1121.
47. Fintel DJ. Antiplatelet therapy in cerebrovascular disease: implications of Management of Artherothrombosis with Clopidogrel in High-risk Patients and the Clopidogrel for High Artherothrombotic Risk and Ischemic Stabilization, Management, and Avoidance studies' results for cardiologists. Clin Cardiol 2007; 30:604–614.
48. Biessels GJ, Luchsinger JA (eds.). Diabetes and the Brain. New York: Humana Press, 2010.
49. Treede RD, Jensen TS, Campbell JN, et al. Neuropathic pain: redefinition and a grading system for clinical and research purposes. Neurology 2008; 70:1630–1635.
50. Gilron I, Bailey JM, Tu D, et al. Morphine, gabapentin, or their combination for neuropathic pain. N Engl J Med 2005; 352:1324–1334.
51. Gilron I, Max MB. Combination pharmacotherapy for neuropathic pain: current evidence and future directions. Expert Rev Neurother 2005; 5:823–830.
52. Melzack R. The McGill Pain Questionnaire: major properties and scoring methods. Pain 1975; 1:277–299.
53. Huskisson EC. Measurement of pain. J Rheumatol 1982; 9:768–769.
54. Cleeland CS, Ryan KM. Pain assessment: global use of the Brief Pain Inventory. Ann Acad Med Singapore 1994; 23:129–138.
55. Gilron I, Watson CP, Cahill CM, et al. Neuropathic pain: a practical guide for the clinician. CMAJ 2006; 175:265–275.
56. Moulin DE, Clark AJ, Gilron I, et al. Pharmacological management of chronic neuropathic pain—consensus statement and guidelines from the Canadian Pain Society. Pain Res Manag 2007; 12:13–21.

57. Dyck PJ, Kratz KM, Karnes JL, et al. The prevalence by staged severity of various types of diabetic neuropathy, retinopathy, and nephropathy in a population-based cohort: The Rochester Diabetic Neuropathy Study. Neurology 1993; 43:817–824.

58. Rundles RW. Diabetic Neuropathy—general review with report of 125 cases. Medicine 1945; 24:111–160.

59. Abbott CA, Carrington AL, Ashe H, et al. The North-West Diabetes Foot Care Study: incidence of, and risk factors for, new diabetic foot ulceration in a community-based patient cohort. Diabet Med 2002; 19:377–384.

60. Chalk C, Benstead TJ, Moore F. Aldose reductase inhibitors for the treatment of diabetic polyneuropathy. Cochrane Database Syst Rev 2007:CD004572.

61. The Diabetes Control and Complications Trial Research Group. The effect of intensive treatment of diabetes on the development and progression of long-term complications in insulin-dependent diabetes mellitus. The Diabetes Control and Complications Trial Research Group. N Engl J Med 1993; 329:977–986.

62. Anonymous. Report and recommendations of the San Antonio conference on diabetic neuropathy. Consensus statement. Diabetes 1988; 37:1000–1004.

63. Bril V, Tomioka S, Buchanan RA, et al. Reliability and validity of the modified Toronto Clinical Neuropathy Score in diabetic sensorimotor polyneuropathy. Diabet Med 2009; 26:240–246.

64. Singleton JR, Bixby B, Russell JW, et al. The Utah Early Neuropathy Scale: a sensitive clinical scale for early sensory predominant neuropathy. J Peripher Nerv Syst 2008; 13:218–227.

65. Feldman EL, Stevens MJ, Thomas PK, et al. A practical two-step quantitative clinical and electrophysiological assessment for the diagnosis and staging of diabetic neuropathy. Diabetes Care 1994; 17:1281–1289.

66. Dyck JB, Dyck PJ. Diabetic polyneuropathy. In: Dyck PJ, Thomas PK, eds. Diabetic Neuropathy. Toronto: W.B. Saunders, 1998:255–278.

67. Dyck PJ, Davies JL, Litchy WJ, et al. Longitudinal assessment of diabetic polyneuropathy using a composite score in the Rochester Diabetic Neuropathy Study cohort. Neurology 1997; 49:229–239.

68. Wilbourn AJ. Diabetic entrapment and compression neuropathies. In: Dyck PJ, Thomas PK, eds. Diabetic Neuropathy. 2nd ed. Toronto: W.B. Saunders, 1999: 481–508.

69. Cook D, Midha R. Meralgia Paresthetica. In: Midha R, Zager EL, eds. Surgery of Peripheral Nerves. New York: Thieme, 2008:167–170.

70. Stewart JD. Focal Peripheral Neuropathies. 4th ed. West Vancouver: JBJ Publishing, 2010.

71. Stewart J. Diabetic truncal neuropathy: topography of the sensory deficit. Ann Neurol 1989; 25:233–238.

72. Raff MC, Sangalang V, Asbury AK. Ischemic mononeuropathy multiplex in association with diabetes mellitus. Neurology 1968; 18:487–499.

73. Morris AM, Deeks SL, Hill MD, et al. Annualized incidence and spectrum of illness from an outbreak investigation of Bell's palsy. Neuroepidemiology 2002; 21:255–261.

74. Barohn RJ, Sahenk Z, Warmolts JR, et al. The Bruns-Garland syndrome (diabetic amyotrophy). Revisited 100 years later. Arch Neurol 1991; 48:1130–1135.

75. Dyck PJ, Windebank AJ. Diabetic and nondiabetic lumbosacral radiculoplexus neuropathies: new insights into pathophysiology and treatment. Muscle Nerve 2002; 25:477–491.

76. Dyck PJ, Norell JE, Dyck PJ. Methylprednisolone may improve lumbosacral radiculoplexus neuropathy. Can J Neurol Sci 2001; 28:224–227.
77. Raff MC, Sangalang V, Asbury AK. Ischemic mononeuropathy multiplex associated with diabetes mellitus. Arch Neurol 1968; 18:487–499.
78. Dyck PJ, Norell JE, Dyck PJ. Microvasculitis and ischemia in diabetic lumbosacral radiculoplexus neuropathy. Neurology 1999; 53:2113–2121.
79. Said G, Elgrably F, Lacroix C, et al. Painful proximal diabetic neuropathy: inflammatory nerve lesions and spontaneous favorable outcome. Ann Neurol 1997; 41:762–770.
80. Neil HA, Thompson AV, John S, et al. Diabetic autonomic neuropathy: the prevalence of impaired heart rate variability in a geographically defined population. Diabet Med 1989; 6:20–24.
81. Veglio M, Sivieri R, Chinaglia A, et al. QT interval prolongation and mortality in type 1 diabetic patients: a 5-year cohort prospective study. Neuropathy Study Group of the Italian Society of the Study of Diabetes, Piemonte Affiliate. Diabetes Care 2000; 23:1381–1383.
82. Bacon CG, Hu FB, Giovannucci E, et al. Association of type and duration of diabetes with erectile dysfunction in a large cohort of men. Diabetes Care 2002; 25:1458–1463.
83. NIH Consensus Conference. Impotence. NIH Consensus Development Panel on Impotence. JAMA 1993; 270:83–90.
84. Watkins PJ. Facial sweating after food: a new sign of diabetic autonomic neuropathy. Br Med J 1973; 1:583–587.
85. Zochodne DW, Kihara M. The autonomic nervous system. In: Brown WF, Bolton CF, eds. Clinical Electromyography. 2nd ed. Toronto: Butterworth-Heinemann, 1993:149–173.
86. Ewing DJ. Which battery of cardiovascular autonomic function tests? Diabetologia 1990; 33:180–181.
87. Ewing DJ, Clarke BF. Diagnosis and management of diabetic autonomic neuropathy. Br Med J 1982; 285:916–918.
88. Kahn R. Proceedings of a consensus development conference on standardized measures in diabetic neuropathy. Autonomic nervous system testing. Diabetes Care 1992; 15:1095–1103.
89. Fealey RD. Thermoregulatory Sweat Test. In: Low PA, ed. Clinical Autonomic Disorders. 2nd ed. Philadelphia: Lippincott-Raven, 1997:245–257.
90. Kennedy WR, Sakuta M, Sutherland D, et al. Quantitation of the sweating deficiency in diabetes mellitus. Ann Neurol 1984; 15:482–488.
91. Gibbons CH, Illigens BM, Wang N, et al. Quantification of sweat gland innervation: a clinical-pathologic correlation. Neurology 2009; 72:1479–1486.
92. Quattrini C, Jeziorska M, Tavakoli M, et al. The Neuropad test: a visual indicator test for human diabetic neuropathy. Diabetologia 2008; 51:1046–1050.
93. Low PA (ed.). Clinical Autonomic Disorders. 2nd ed. Philadelphia: Lippincott-Raven, 1997.
94. Petersen RC, Stevens JC, Ganguli M, et al. Practice parameter: early detection of dementia: mild cognitive impairment (an evidence-based review). Report of the Quality Standards Subcommittee of the American Academy of Neurology Neurology 2001; 56:1133–1142.

95. Schneider JA, Arvanitakis Z, Bang W, et al. Mixed brain pathologies account for most dementia cases in community-dwelling older persons. Neurology 2007; 69:2197–2204.
96. Seshadri S, Wolf PA. Lifetime risk of stroke and dementia: current concepts, and estimates from the Framingham Study. Lancet Neurol 2007; 6:1106–1114.
97. Biessels GJ, Staekenborg S, Brunner E, et al. Risk of dementia in diabetes mellitus: a systematic review. Lancet Neurol 2006; 5:64–74.
98. Weuve J, McQueen MB, Blacker D. The AlzRisk Database, 2010.
99. Schmahmann JD, Smith EE, Eichler FS, et al. Cerebral white matter: neuro-anatomy, clinical neurology, and neurobehavioral correlates. Ann N Y Acad Sci 2008; 1142:266–309.
100. Vermeer SE, Prins ND, den HT, et al. Silent brain infarcts and the risk of dementia and cognitive decline. N Engl J Med 2003; 348:1215–1222.
101. Qiu WQ, Folstein MF. Insulin, insulin-degrading enzyme and amyloid-beta peptide in Alzheimer's disease: review and hypothesis. Neurobiol Aging 2006; 27:190–198.
102. Peila R, Rodriguez BL, Launer LJ. Type 2 diabetes, APOE gene, and the risk for dementia and related pathologies: the Honolulu-Asia Aging Study. Diabetes 2002; 51:1256–1262.
103. Doody RS, Stevens JC, Beck C, et al. Practice parameter: management of dementia (an evidence-based review). Report of the Quality Standards Subcommittee of the American Academy of Neurology. Neurology 2001; 56:1154–1166.
104. Hogan DB, Bailey P, Black S, et al. Diagnosis and treatment of dementia: 4. approach to management of mild to moderate dementia. CMAJ 2008; 179:787–793.
105. Hogan DB, Bailey P, Black S, et al. Diagnosis and treatment of dementia: nonpharmacologic and pharmacologic therapy for mild to moderate dementia. CMAJ 2008; 179:1019–1026.
106. Herrmann N, Gauthier S. Diagnosis and treatment of dementia: 6. Management of severe Alzheimer disease. CMAJ 2008; 179:1279–1287.
107. Scottish Intercollegiate Guidelines Network (SIGN). Management of patients with dementia. A national clinical guideline, 2006.
108. Waldemar G, Dubois B, Emre M, et al. Recommendations for the diagnosis and management of Alzheimer's disease and other disorders associated with dementia: EFNS guideline. Eur J Neurol 2007; 14:e1–e26.
109. Singh S, Wooltorton E. Increased mortality among elderly patients with dementia using atypical antipsychotics. CMAJ 2005; 173:252.
110. Plassman BL, Langa KM, Fisher GG, et al. Prevalence of dementia in the United States: the aging, demographics, and memory study. Neuroepidemiology 2007; 29:125–132.
111. Rajagopalan S. Serious infections in elderly patients with diabetes mellitus. Clin Infect Dis 2005; 40:990–996.
112. Torre-Cisneros J, Lopez OL, Kusne S, et al. CNS aspergillosis in organ trans-plantation: a clinicopathological study. J Neurol Neurosurg Psychiatry 1993; 56:188–193.
113. Norlinah MI, Ngow HA, Hamidon BB. Angioinvasive cerebral aspergillosis presenting as acute ischaemic stroke in a patient with diabetes mellitus. Singapore Med J 2007; 48:e1–e4.
114. Reihsaus E, Waldbaur H, Seeling W. Spinal epidural abscess: a meta-analysis of 915 patients. Neurosurg Rev 2000; 23:175–204.

115. Cascio A, Stassi G, Costa GB, et al. Chryseobacterium indologenes bacteraemia in a diabetic child. J Med Microbiol 2005; 54:677–680.
116. Bader MS. Diabetic foot infection. Am Fam Physician 2008; 78:71–79.
117. Peleg AY, Weerarathna T, McCarthy JS, et al. Common infections in diabetes: pathogenesis, management and relationship to glycaemic control. Diabetes Metab Res Rev 2007; 23:3–13.
118. Bolton CF, McKeown MJ, Chen R, et al. Subacute uremic and diabetic polyneuropathy. Muscle Nerve 1997; 20:59–64.
119. Bolton CF, Remtulla H, Toth B, et al. Distinctive electrophysiological features of denervated muscle in uremic patients. J Clin Neurophysiol 1997; 14:539–542.
120. Bolton CF, Driedger AA, Lindsay RM. Ischaemic neuropathy in uraemic patients caused by bovine arteriovenous shunt. J Neurol Neurosurg Psychiatry 1979; 42:810–814.
121. Bolton CF, Young GB. Neurological Complications of Renal Disease. Boston: Butterworths, 1990.
122. Bolton CF, Baltzan MA, Baltzan RB. Effects of renal transplantation on uremic neuropathy. A clinical and electrophysiologic study. N Engl J Med 1971; 284:1170–1175.
123. Cotton F, Kamoun S, Rety-Jacob F, et al. Acute hypertensive encephalopathy with widespread small-vessel disease at MRI in a diabetic patient: pathogenetic hypotheses. Neuroradiology 2005; 47:599–603.
124. Servillo G, Bifulco F, De Robertis, et al. Posterior reversible encephalopathy syndrome in intensive care medicine. Intensive Care Med 2007; 33:230–236.
125. Ropper AH. Accelerated neuropathy of renal failure. Arch Neurol 1993; 50:536–539.
126. Ganie MA, Bhat D. Current developments in Wolfram syndrome. J Pediatr Endocrinol Metab 2009; 22:3–10.
127. Hilson JB, Merchant SN, Adams JC, et al. Wolfram syndrome: a clinicopathologic correlation. Acta Neuropathol 2009; 118:415–428.
128. Sproule DM, Kaufmann P. Mitochondrial encephalopathy, lactic acidosis, and strokelike episodes: basic concepts, clinical phenotype, and therapeutic management of MELAS syndrome. Ann N Y Acad Sci 2008; 1142:133–158.
129. Ristow M. Neurodegenerative disorders associated with diabetes mellitus. J Mol Med 2004; 82:510–529.
130. Perseghin G, Caumo A, Arcelloni C, et al. Contribution of abnormal insulin secretion and insulin resistance to the pathogenesis of type 2 diabetes in myotonic dystrophy. Diabetes Care 2003; 26:2112–2118.
131. Resmini E, Minuto F, Colao A, et al. Secondary diabetes associated with principal endocrinopathies: the impact of new treatment modalities. Acta Diabetol 2009; 46:85–95.
132. Schulz JB, Boesch S, Burk K, et al. Diagnosis and treatment of Friedreich ataxia: a European perspective. Nat Rev Neurol 2009; 5:222–234.
133. Gandhi GY, Basu R, Dispenzieri A, et al. Endocrinopathy in POEMS syndrome: the Mayo Clinic experience. Mayo Clin Proc 2007; 82:836–842.
134. Pober BR. Williams-Beuren syndrome. N Engl J Med 2010; 362:239–252.
135. Tatum WO, Passaro EA, Elia M, et al. Seizures in Klinefelter's syndrome. Pediatr Neurol 1998; 19:275–278.
136. Wattendorf DJ, Muenke M. Klinefelter syndrome. Am Fam Physician 2005; 72:2259–2262.

Index